Hands on Health

Holistic Healing

The Whole Food Kitchen Series

Hands On Health

*Take Your Vibrant, Whole Health
Back Into Your Healing Hands*

Paula M. Youmell, RN, MS, CHC
Certified Holistic Health Counselor

Foreword: Shelby Connelly, L.Ac.

Five Elements Living Wellness Retreat Center

BALBOA.
PRESS
A DIVISION OF HAY HOUSE

Balboa Press books may be ordered through booksellers or by contacting:

Balboa Press
A Division of Hay House
1663 Liberty Drive
Bloomington, IN 47403
www.balboapress.com
1-(877) 407-4847

Printed in the United States of America

ISBN: 978-1-4525-6590-3 (sc)
ISBN: 978-1-4525-6592-7 (hc)
ISBN: 978-1-4525-6591-0 (e)

Library of Congress Control Number: 2012924003

Balboa Press rev. date: 3/28/2013

Dedication

To my Grampa, Myron Youmell, my first teacher in the art of natural healing and herbal medicine. I am grateful for the many times I watched you stir your herbal brews and strain them into your brown bottles. Your kitchen "magic" stirred the part of me that knows healing comes from within, from nature.

To my Grams, Katherine Page and Marion Youmell, and my Grampa, Glenn Page, who taught me that healing ourselves was best kept in our own hands.

To my parents, Francis and Glenda (Page) Youmell, for continuing the reminder that health and healing are innate in us and bringing me up to know I can do anything I set myself to.

To Jake and Eli,

My inspirations

An apple a day keeps the doctor away

Origin: Wales

The February 1866 edition of *Notes and Queries* magazine includes this:

"A Pembrokeshire proverb. Eat an apple on going to bed, and you'll keep the doctor from earning his bread."

http://www.phrases.org.uk

APPLE LOVE

To spread a little "apple love" in the world; proceeds from this book will be used to support my favorite, local non-profits:

Little River Community School www.littleriverschool.org

GardenShare www.gardenshare.org

The Sustainable Living Project www.sustainablelivingproject.net

These agencies support:

Healthy, happy kids who learn through love,

Whole foods grown locally,

Rural and sustainable living skills for a better community -- micro and macro!

Table of Contents

Foreword

Shelby Connelly, L.Ac.
www.fiveelementsliving.com

THE FIRST YEAR I OPENED my practice I met Paula Youmell. She called seeking acupuncture and asked how it could help her fine tune her own health. On her very first treatment we became fast friends. Her scheduled treatments weren't nearly enough time for us to talk about the thousands of health-related topics we wanted to cover. It was so refreshing to find a practitioner with a Western medical background so deeply imbedded in Eastern philosophy. I had struck GOLD! Not only has she guided me with coaching patients, she has helped me tremendously with my own wellness, seen me through personal struggles, and been my touchstone on the health choices I've made for my children.

I have been a holistic practitioner for over 15 years and I am still amazed at how my patients view their own health and wellness. Whether it is chronic or acute physical or emotional pain, many have the mindset that their dis-ease* is out of their control. They come with stories of disappointment and despair from not being able to find hope in a quick fix or a magic pill. When they arrive at my door they are looking for a magic needle. Since I became an acupuncturist, I too, have been searching for answers. Not answers on how to fix what is already broken but how can I achieve optimal wellness and keep it. I wanted to empower my patients and teach them that the control over their health is their own. Over the past 14 years I have found answers through Paula. She

*Dis-ease: lack of ease in the body, the origin of disease.

has taught me to look at the body as a garden, not a machine, and has inspired me to think in ways of tending and nurturing and not fixing and mending.

We are at constant war with our bodies: asking them to function at optimum capacity without optimal care. I include myself in the "we," as I am well versed through Paula's guidance yet constantly refocusing on the task at hand. I can relate to my dear patients. I understand the wanting to push my body and spirit harder than I give it the tools to succeed. Paula has taught me the practice--as it is a practice--of giving daily, sometimes hourly, care to myself. Paula teaches common sense, the basics yet so deeply foreign in our culture. She teaches us the ease of self-care, making it accessible to every human being.

While acupuncture, chiropractic, physical therapy, massage, and even surgery can help clear the path to better observation of ourselves--it is the on- going, daily practice of tending to our bodies that will keep us well. The lessons Paula creates can put us beyond weight loss, above "all right" and further into our intended life span. This book will inspire you to find your own power to heal!

My Preface

I WRITE THIS BOOK TO remind everyone of their own innate ability to heal. Healing is the norm. If you cut your finger, it heals without intervention. Every part of your body is capable of healing if it is given what it needs to heal and thrive. This is a Vitalist philosophy of healing: Healing comes through nature. You **are** nature; therefore, healing comes from within you and through you.

Despite longer life spans, people are not necessarily living healthier lives. Much of our older years are plagued with disease symptoms that are managed and squelched by prescription medications and other medical treatments that do not actually invoke real healing.

People say all the time, "My grandfather lived to be 89, so we must be doing something right with health care." Chances are that grandparent grew up on food raised naturally in the backyard garden and barnyard or by the farmer down the street. Even people living in urban areas were being fed by farmers growing whole foods close by the city. When a body is built from conception on (and this really goes back through generations of good whole food living, passing strong cellular health to the next generation) with whole foods, the body grows up with intact, whole cellular health. Each generation of cell reproduction was created with whole foods growing up a body on a solid foundation of good, healthy cells.

Our increased longevity can also be attributed to better sanitation, use of antibiotics (unfortunately, we are now paying for the overuse of them), and easier lifestyles. The hard labor and constant exposure to the elements, in those generations living and working more closely to the land, were factors in earlier death. If we look at colonial days, wealthy land owners lived longer lives (if they did not contract an infectious disease and not recover from it) than the field hands working the land, constantly exposed to hard physical labor and the elements.

When we look at children growing up in today's fast food and "food product" culture, we are seeing different results. As their bodies grow and develop from their conception on with packaged, refined foods being a staple of the diet, we are witnessing the new generation of humans who have degenerative diseases at very early ages. Children and teenagers are developing type 2, adult onset diabetes, high blood pressure, high cholesterol, and cardiovascular disease. I think this speaks loudly about our cultural movement away from traditional eating of whole, well-raised food to a culture of packaged, processed "food products." Our cultural cellular health and integrity are suffering.

I offer this book as a simple reminder of health and healing, a simple solution to the symptoms that bother you. What I write in this book is what I have found to be truths--truths for me, based upon my learning, experience, and resultant wisdom (or so called wisdom). As you read, question everything. Avoid being a passive sponge soaking up the information I lay out for you. Question and seek your own answers. Create your own truths.

My own interest in healing began in my first year of nursing school. I watched how patients were cared for in the hospitals. Their symptoms were "managed," but people were never helped to heal, never reminded of what we intuitively know. Healing can and will happen.

Thus began a 25 year journey learning about nutrition, herbs, energy, emotional and spiritual health, and healing. May the health and healing path I have walked make your path to health and healing much shorter.

Writer's Waiver: I write this book from the information in my head; you will not find a bibliography or footnotes. I have used my educational and real life experience as a registered nurse, school health and physical education teacher, yoga practitioner and teacher, herbalist, reiki practitioner, and whole food educator. I added the many dashes of the wisdom I have gained through my holistic trainings under naturopaths, herbalists, energy healers, and many other natural healers, as well as the common sense that becomes inherent in working with the natural balance of life.

Please relax and enjoy our healing conversation.

Thanks and Praise

I THANK ALL THE NATURAL healers who have shared their knowledge, wisdom, and healing skills and have inspired me to delve deeper into what is our healing heritage: Dr. John Christopher, Dr. Richard Schulze, Rosemary Gladstar, James Green, Susun Weed, Dr. Andrew Weil, Lillian Casserly, Shelby Connelly, Helen Kenny, Joshua Rosenthal, Dianne Fineout, and so many more!

Special thanks to:

Jake and Eli for the use of their precious hands in the cover photo. Jake for the cover photo editing and both boys for their unconditional love and tolerance of Mom's unending quest for their holistic health.

Shelby Connelly for being my friend, mentor, co-conspirator in health, and for writing the foreword words of wisdom.

Bob Zywicki, an average Joe with regard to health information (though as a human being, by no means an average Joe!) for taking on the job of editing my book for content, clarity, flow of thoughts, and general ability to educate and inspire others towards health and healing. You are awesome, Bob!

Kelly Burnham, my editor in chief, for her hard work fine-tooth combing my manuscript. You are amazing, Kelly, and I thank you from the bottom of my heart.

Ginny, my sister, for being behind me as I do what I do, twisting Bob's arm to edit (how hard **did** you twist?), and always seeming to remember when I have big events happening and sending words of encouragement.

Terry, my sister, for being a grounded human being. I tend to be someone who takes "the leap" into new adventures and only *then* do I look to see where I am actually jumping. Terry is my role model of stability.

Jay for cooperating with my holistic mothering and for co-creating Jakob and Eli, our life's treasures.

Michele Smith of Forever Fit With Michele, Anti-Aging Specialist, Nutritionist, Fitness Coach, NYC. Thanks for being a wise and inspiring mentor. www.foreverfitwithmichele.com

Scott Miller, former manager of the Potsdam Food Coop for being the instigator of my health and healing writing passion.

Carol Pynchon for the initial editing advice.

Balboa Press for their awesome help in my self-publishing endeavor: Andrea Geasey (thanks for keeping me motivated!) and Stephanie Cornthwaite for all your help.

A special thanks to all of my clients and students, over the years, who have taught me:

> **My way, being the right way for me in any given moment, is not always "the" way for them,**
>
> **Never give up on anyone. What inspires change is not always what I expect it to be, and**
>
> **Do the best you can in any and every given moment.**
>
> **Thanks for trusting me to walk with you on your path to health.**

Disclaimer

YOUR HEALTH IS YOUR RESPONSIBILITY, plain and simple. Any information in this book is for you to use as you see fit on your path to health and healing. The author and publisher are not responsible for choices you make regarding your health. Information contained within these pages is meant to educate and inform you so you can invoke self-responsibility and take your health into your own healing hands. Take what I have learned about nutrition, health, and healing and create your own healing truths.

Walk with peace and love on your path to health and healing.

Blessings, Paula

Self-Responsibility

Health is about self-responsibility. Taking your health into your own hands is what Hands On Health is about. The ability to heal lies within us. The responsibility to care for our bodies to ensure lifelong health, prevent disease and heal lies within us. Healers are those people, including our own selves, who walk with us on our path to mind, body, and spiritual health and healing.

So many clients tell me, "Oh, I can't do this; I can't give up my
_____."

Whole Health Healing is not about what you are giving up, it is not about deprivation. It **IS** about what you are inviting into your life: the choices, changes, and additions that will open doors to healing, health, and happiness in ways you have never imagined or experienced.

Be brave. Take that first step on your own healing path, knowing every new step will be an adventure and a positive, healing challenge. **Wherever you are in your life, however long you have been taking less that "whole" care of your body, every step you take towards whole foods and whole health living will make lasting changes in your cellular and whole body health.**

I bold faced the above sentence because Bob, my content editor, asked me this about the information in this book: "Am I too late?" "If someone has *poisoned* their body for many years, perhaps decades, of unhealthy eating and lifestyle choices, is there any hope for them?" I will repeat this throughout the book: every step you take towards whole foods and whole health living will make lasting changes in your cellular and whole body health. **No, it is not too late, and yes, there is much hope! Jumpstart your health now!**

Walk lightly on your path!

Chapter 1
Whole Health

"We cannot solve our problems with the same level of thinking that created them"
Albert Einstein

HEALTH IS A PERSON'S STATE of wholeness of mind, body and spirit. This state of wholeness fluctuates as we move through our days and our life. Health does not mean you are without symptoms. You can live in whole health, co-existing with your symptoms, making the best of every day. The lifestyle choices we make daily walk our body either in the direction of health and healing or towards symptoms and diseases.

Our current health care system does not work with the wholeness of health, the wholeness of individuals. Truly, it is a disease care system where problems are taken care of at the end stage, when the body has already broken down. You are medically treated with drugs, surgery, chemotherapy, etc. to turn off the symptoms presented. This is much like cutting the wire to your cars *check engine* light. You have rid your car of the symptom, the warning light, but you have not solved the problem.

True "health care" IS about promoting whole health, preventing the breakdown of healthy bodies and truly healing when symptoms appear. It is not about merely covering up and extinguishing symptoms of ill health and disease. Symptoms are your warning light. Taking your health into your own hands, exercising self-responsibility for your health means figuring out the cause(s) of your symptoms and removing these causes from your life.

When we remove the cause of disease, the body can begin its natural healing process. Then we can cleanse the causes of symptoms and work to nourish and rebuild the body back to whole health.

Healing, returning the body to whole health, takes time. If creating the symptoms of disease has taken a long time to appear, have patience and your body will heal. Quick fixes, silver bullets to health and healing, do not exist. Health and healing are a long-term commitment for you. A wise healer once told me to expect one month of healing for every year it took to create disease.

Patience heals. Have faith in your innate, natural capacity to heal.

> *"Many things which cannot be overcome when they are together,*
> *yield themselves up when taken little by little."*
>
> **Plutarch**

You are a Micro of the Macro

The human body **is** a microcosm of the macrocosm. The macrocosm being Earth!

Think about how your body is comparable to the Earth as a whole:

- The blood running through your arteries and veins is like Earth's waters running through the rivers and streams.
- The extracellular fluid - the fluid surrounding and bathing your cells - is like the swamp land of our earth's rivers and streams. Swamp land is an exchange area between the rivers, streams, and the dry land beyond the swamp. Extracellular fluid is the exchange area between cells.
- Your tissues are like the soil of the Earth.

"Man did not weave the web of life; he is merely a strand in it. Whatever he does to the web, he does to himself. "

Chief Seattle

A modern translation:

"What we do to the Earth, we do to ourselves."

Isabel Clarke

Your body is truly a microcosm of the Earth, the macrocosm. When you care for the Earth, you care for yourself and all life on this planet. When you keep the Earth's waterways, soil and air clean; you keep your cells, tissues, and organs clean.

What befalls the Earth befalls humans!

Let's take care of ourselves, the living beings around us, and our home - the Earth - in a holistic, whole health manner.

The following Chapters have been written, with simplicity and light-hearted fun, to help guide you in making whole health choices to prevent disease, heal symptoms, and live a vibrant, whole health life.

The bottom line: Do the best you can every day to eat whole food and live a whole health lifestyle. Be kind to yourself in every moment knowing you are being your best self for this moment. Each day is a moment for new beginnings, new possibilities with no guilt and no regrets.

Please read on to open your awareness, your true self, to whole food eating and whole health living. **Every little step you make to change your lifestyle will have paybacks in your body's health and healing whether you are two or 82 years old.**

Chapter 2
Principles of Whole Food Nutrition

"Let food be thy medicine, let medicine be thy food."

Hippocrates

WHOLE FOOD EATING MEANS FEEDING our bodies the way nature intended. This means eating foods in their natural state, as close to the perfectly "whole" state in which nature provides them. This also means following the natural growing seasons and eating more foods that are locally grown and produced.

Whole food nutrition is eating in balance, which in turn keeps your body's health balanced. Foods grown naturally develop with the right proportion of carbohydrates, proteins, and fats intended for that particular food. They contain balanced vitamins, minerals, phyto-nutrients, and enzymes. This natural balance for each food ensures that the body can properly utilize the nutrients. Foods that have been refined or processed (parts of them removed or altered) or enriched/fortified (things added) upset this natural balance in food. Food that has been altered will upset the natural balance of your body.

The effects of moving away from whole foods and towards refined, processed and convenience foods are very prevalent in our society. Cancer, cardiovascular, bone, teeth, weight, and many other health problems are directly related to this change to our "modern" diet. Traditional societies, who still eat whole foods, suffer very minimally from these health problems. As a society, we spend much time looking for cures. The cure is most often in the prevention. The return to whole health is simple: make the choice to return to whole food principles of eating and whole health lifestyle choices.

"Men dig their graves with their own teeth and die more by those fated instruments than all the weapons of their enemies."

Thomas Moffett, 1600 AD

"The cure is the same as the prevention. Let food be thy medicine."

Hippocrates

On a very simple level, anyone can tell that a baked or steamed, whole potato is more nutritious than potato chips. When you use that thought process with every food choice your health improves. Ask yourself, "How close is this food to its natural, whole state?" This question makes it very obvious what food should be included and what food should be excluded from our daily fare.

The following grouping of whole foods will get you started on the whole food nutrition concept:

Vegetables: Buy fresh, seasonal produce (better yet, grow as much as you can of your own food or make friends with farmers who grow it for you) and eat it as whole as possible: raw or very lightly steamed. Lightly steamed means vegetables should retain their color and crisp texture, 2 to 3 minutes for small vegetables and greens, and slightly more time for larger vegetables. Soups and stews in the winter are cooked longer and slower to nourish you in cold weather.

Fruit: Raw is best. Dried, frozen, and canned, local fruit is good during the off-season. Eat dried fruit in moderation. It is a concentrated sugar source. Frozen is better than canned. Fruit juices are merely liquid fruit sugar and are best avoided. Opt to eat the whole fruit. (Juice fasting is another book!)

Beans and Legumes: Fresh, in season is best; very good raw and lightly steamed. Dried beans, in the off season, are a nutritious source of protein, vitamins, and minerals. It is an enjoyable art form learning how to cook and create meals with them: soups, dips, sandwich spreads, casseroles, bean milks, bean burgers and loafs, hearty additions to breads/muffins/cookies -- the list is inexhaustible. Try sprouting for added nutrition. Sprouting of some beans makes them enjoyable in the raw, sprouted state. Other beans are not edible in the sprouted state until you cook them. Cooking time is much less for sprouted beans, which is an extended soak process.

Nuts and Seeds: Whole and raw is best with most nuts and seeds. Raw nut butters are a delicious and fun alternative. Raw peanuts and peanut butter are not recommended. Eat both roasted. Peanuts are actually legumes/beans. Nuts and seeds are a good source of healthy fat; just remember to eat in moderation.

Grains: Learn to cook and enjoy whole grains: oats, rye, millet, rice, kamut, buckwheat, teff, wheat berries, barley, quinoa, spelt, corn, and amaranth. They can all be cooked and eaten like whole grain brown rice and enjoyed cold in salads, hot in soups/casseroles/pilafs. Cooked whole grains are tasty hot cereals or use dinner leftovers as cold cereal. Mix the leftovers with plain yogurt, nuts and seeds, cinnamon, vanilla, and a touch of raw honey or maple syrup. Maple syrup may not be a locally available sweetener for you. Seek out the whole food sweeteners that are traditionally used in your geographic area.

When choosing flour and flour products (breads, pastas, pastries, cookies and baked goods) make certain that all flours used in the products are **100% whole grains**. Avoid the refined, bleached, enriched, unbleached, all-purpose and cake flours. Better yet, make your own flour products if you can. That way you are in total control of all your baking ingredients being whole foods. Grains are easy to grind into flour in a high-quality blender or grinder made for this purpose.

All of the above grains can be ground into flour. If you play in the kitchen with recipes, you will figure out which whole grain flours work best for different foods. I like spelt and oat flour for cookies and cakes. I will also use corn, teff, amaranth, quinoa, and buckwheat flours. Remember to try all of these whole food flours when making the whole food treat recipes in Chapter 10.

Nuts such as almonds, hazelnuts, and coconut can also be ground into flour and used to replace grain flours. Many people do better, health and weight wise, keeping the grains to a minimum in their diet. Grains are used to fatten cattle and life stock — need I say more?

Fats and Oils: Your healthiest option is fats from whole foods, not oils. All of the above whole foods contain varying amounts of fat. The foods listed below contain high percentages of healthy fat and should be eaten in moderation. Getting healthy fat from whole foods means making choices like these:

- Sesame seeds or tahini, not sesame oil
- Almonds or almond butter, not almond oil
- Olives, not olive oil
- Flax seeds, not flax seed oil
- Avocados, not avocado oil
- Fermented soy foods, not soy oil

When oils are used, make **certain** you are buying high quality **cold pressed** oils, not refined, chemically extracted oils. Most supermarket oils are poor quality and chemically extracted. Cold pressed is more expensive, but remember your health is worth it. Think preventive maintenance, restorative health and healing!

My favorite cooking oil is sesame, some people enjoy coconut oil. Both hold out well to the heat of normal cooking. I truly prefer a good quality, grass-fed butter for cooking and baking. I use extra virgin olive oil for raw purposes: homemade salad dressings and splashing on vegetables. If you prefer, as I do, let grass-fed butter melt on cooked vegetables!

Fish: Fish caught in the wild or naturally raised fish are a good source of protein and fat. Avoid fish raised in fish farms. Fish raised in farms are fed unnatural diets of manufactured *pellet food*. They are given antibiotics to combat diseases acquired from living in close quarters and unnatural conditions (much like factory farm raised animals). Naturally raised means the fish are eating the same foods they would eat in the wild.

Animal Products: This includes meats, poultry, eggs, milk, and dairy products. Buy products from animals fed naturally and raised free range. Organically, free-range raised is even better. Example: cows who graze and eat natural grasses, not grain fed cows. Natural lifestyles ensure animal products that are lower in saturated fat and high in health-promoting omega-3 fats.

If an animal is raised in a natural, healthy manner the animal products will be naturally balanced and healthy for consumption. Think about eating wild fish. Wild fish create healthy fats and proteins because they are eating their natural, whole foods and living a natural, whole health lifestyle. If fish can accomplish a personal healthy fat ratio by eating their natural diet obviously other animals do too. Fish do not have some magical ability that no other creature on earth has!

This is about your cell biology. If you eat a diet that is 100% whole foods and those foods were raised naturally, your body cells are healthy. When organisms live a whole health lifestyle the result is whole beings. It is that simple.

On the other hand, if animals are fed unhealthy and un-natural foods the animal will be unhealthy. Think about what happens to humans who feed themselves unhealthy and unnatural food. I am referring to that cell reproduction, the cell biology lesson down a few paragraphs. The body cells of animals, being fed un-natural diets, degenerate. Their bodies become unhealthy when they are fed un-natural diets. Eating the resultant animal products is not going to be a health promoting choice for you.

Unwrapping Butter's Bad Rap

The information below is going to fly in the face of everything you have "learned" about cholesterol. Take a deep breath when you read it and let your common sense prevail. Think about Native Americans, did they shun animal fat? How about the Inuit Eskimos who lived on whale flesh and blubber? Not a chance! Traditional people gobbled up the fat knowing it held amazing life giving energy and nutrients.

As soon as animals birth their offspring, their mammary glands roll into production and milk (a life sap) becomes plentiful. Along with milk comes cream, the precursor to one of my favorite condiments -- butter: yummy, sweet cream butter!

Over the years, butter has been given a bad rap. Just what is said about butter (and fats in general) and how much truth is in this information? Butter has been blamed for cardiac disease and all the symptoms leading up to it (high cholesterol, high blood pressure, etc.), cancer, and a host of other symptoms that get compiled together into various diseases.

I have many questions surrounding this information:

1. Are saturated fats really bad for human health?

2. How does the quality of the animals' food and lifestyle affect their health? Does their health, or lack of it, affect your health when you eat their products?

3. How healthy are synthetically produced saturated fats: hydrogenated oils, margarine?

4. Which is healthier: animal or plant fats?

5. What is the logic behind the warning: "fats that are solid at room temperature should never be eaten"?

Back to butter and saturated fats for thoughts on question #1. Saturated fat is needed by the body for:

- endorphin and neurotransmitter production
- fat soluble vitamin absorption, metabolism, and usage of omega 3 fats
- eye health and prevention of macular degeneration
- proper function of the thyroid and bodily metabolism
- healthy cell membranes
- incorporation of calcium into your skeleton for the formation and maintenance of healthy bones
- protection of liver from toxins such as alcohol, prescription, and OTC medications
- immune system enhancement
- hormone production and fertility enhancement

"Saturated fat is not the root of all evil … and it is not to blame for the modern disease epidemics facing Americans. Saturated fat is actually an incredibly healthy, nourishing and all natural fat that humans have been thriving on for generations." Quote from Sally Fallon and Mary Enig, leading researchers and nutritional experts who wrote the book *Nourishing Traditions: The Cookbook that Challenges Politically Correct Nutrition and the Diet Dictocrats.*

Where did the idea that saturated fats are bad begin? In 1953, Dr. Ancel Key published a paper on fat intake and heart disease. His research analysis and findings have since been proven flawed. However, in the 1950's his theories linking animal fats to heart disease caught on quickly and persist today. Most people refuse to let go of the theory that butter is bad for us, clogging our arteries and creating disease.

Margarine* (hydrogenated**, artificially flavored vegetable oils) was introduced to our food culture in the late 1800's. It was marketed as a much healthier alternative to butter because it was from plant-based oils. Margarine was widely distributed during WWII and then a decade or so later Key's "research" pushed margarine's popularity even further.

Butter is a naturally occurring saturated fat. Because of butter's saturated state, it resists going rancid much longer than liquid, veggie oils. Hydrogenated oils were created to mimic butter's ability to resist going rancid but at grave consequences to the health of those who eat the hydrogenated fats.

My thoughts on the above questions #2, 3 and 4:

I have my own theories, formulated over my years working in natural health. Any food - plant or animal based - if raised 100% naturally, just

*Margarine:** Originally developed by a French chemist in the late 19th century, margarine was created in response to a request from the French government to invent a cheap, long, shelf-life butter substitute that could feed its armies on the march.

Hydrogenated and partially hydrogenated oils are created by adding hydrogen bonds to the chemical structure of the plant oil. This process saturates the available bonds of the molecule. The end result is a solid fat produced from naturally occurring liquid oil. This synthetic saturation serves a purpose in the food manufacturing world. Hydrogenation makes vegetable oils more stable and extends the shelf life of products containing these hydrogenated oils. These synthetic saturated fats contain trans fats. Trans fats are a major health problem. They are synthetic fats that wreak havoc on human health.

as it would grow and mature on its own, without human intervention, can only be nourishing to our bodies. Nature intended this! When humans start interrupting natural processes - feeding plants and animals unnatural substances and forcing them to live unnatural lifestyles - their products become unhealthy for other organisms to eat.

Butter, from animals naturally fed and cared for, contains a balanced array of essential fatty acids and nutrients. This means your health (and the health of animals producing the products) would be best served if we choose to eat dairy products from grass-fed, not grain-fed animals. Turn that grass-fed cream into butter and its natural array of fats will be used for all the fat needs of your body. (Please refer to the above uses of saturated fats in the human body.)

Specific blessings of butter from grass-fed animals:

- rich source of easily absorbable vitamin A
- good source of all fat soluble vitamins
- rich in important trace minerals, high in selenium and iodine
- a perfect blend of fatty acids

I like to compare grass-fed *land* animals to the "eat wild fish" agenda that has been popular for some time. You are told how the fats in wild Alaskan salmon and other deep, cold-water ocean fish are good for us. Are fish really the only animals that can eat their natural diets and turn this food into healthy fat that is good for both the fish's health and for the humans who choose to eat them? It does not make a bit of sense to me that fish are the only living creatures capable of this feat. I believe that all animals, eating their natural diets, uninterrupted by humans' manufactured "food products" are producing 100% healthy bodies, their fat included. **Warning:** farm-raised salmon and other fish are unhealthy. They are fed unnatural diets creating unhealthy bodies with unhealthy fat profiles. Tampering with nature does not pay off!

Grain-fed dairy animals produce cream that is unbalanced in its fatty acid profile. Consuming unbalanced, unhealthy fats from animals (or hydrogenated vegetable fats) will only create chaos and un-health – disease - in the human body.

The question arises: between animal and plant based fats, which one is healthier? I have my thoughts and theories here too. (Bet you are surprised!) If the animals are raised naturally, their fat in moderation is not unhealthy in our diets. Peeling a stick of butter and eating it like a banana, while appealing to some, is NOT moderation!

I will repeat my thoughts here on plant-based fats: they are best in their whole, natural state also: avocados over avocado oil, olives over olive oil, nuts and seeds over their oils. Those plants need to be raised organically and sustainably so they contain the full array of nutrients that nature intended.

Now some thoughts on question # 5:

Average room temperature is somewhere around 60 to 70 degrees F. The average body temperature is a bit higher than that, say somewhere around 98.6 F. Where does that leave solid fats in this huge temperature discrepancy? I have to assume any animal fat that is solid at 60 to 70 degrees is going to look and function a bit differently at 98.6 degrees. I don't know, I could be wrong.

Possible research sites for more information:

- www.westonaprice.org/ (article "Why Butter is Better")
- www.eatwild.com
- www.americangrassfed.com
- www.raw-milk-facts.com/raw_milk_health_benefits.html
- www.realmilk.com

Paula M. Youmell, RN, MS, CHC

Writer's Disclaimer: The writer's knowledge and experiences are not necessarily shared, nor have they been evaluated or approved by the F.D.A., the A.M.A., or any other agency. My theories, beliefs, and hypotheses come from 20 plus years of studying and working in natural nutrition and healing. Eat butter at your own risk and pleasure - I do!

Bottom Line: Planning your diets with these whole food principles in mind will create health and lifetime wellness. Whole foods and whole health living prevent lifestyle diseases and stimulate healing if a problem already exist.

Note: There is not one diet prescription that works for everyone. Individuals thrive on different percentages of carbohydrates, proteins and fats. Using a 100% whole food diet, based upon what is naturally available locally and seasonally (is butter a naturally/ locally produced food in your area?), discover what works for you and live this whole health lifestyle. Keep in mind your nutritional needs may change with the changing seasons of the year and your life.

Benefits of Whole Food Eating, Whole Health Living

"Eating healthy foods, eating organic foods is just too expensive. How can I afford to eat healthy on my income/budget?" I hear these comments all the time and have for 25 years of working with people and their health. I have to tell you the benefits that come from this healthy lifestyle choice are immeasurable.

The old adage **"an ounce of prevention is worth a pound of cure"** could not ring more true! Let's examine this information together.

Your body cells depend on the food you eat to reproduce, repair, and thrive. Whole foods reproduce whole, healthy cells. Processed, refined package foods and junk fast foods create cells that are degenerated, less healthy than the original parent cell. A lifetime of non-whole food eating and your cells have progressively degenerated many, many times. This is what creates degenerative disease.

Body cells make body tissues, which form body organs. The body organs form organ systems. All the organ systems together create an organism, You! Healthy cellular biology depends on the food you eat and the lifestyle choices you make every day. Your tissues, organs, organ systems, *you* (the organism) can only be as healthy and whole as the foods you eat. That was your basic human biology lesson for the day. Hope you enjoyed it!

Here is another comparison I make for people. If your body were a savings account it would work like this: when you put whole foods into your body, your body recognizes them as natural foods. You digest whole foods with little effort. The nutrients are used for bodily processes and stored in your cells, the body's savings account. When you eat processed, refined foods your body does not recognize and digest them easily. Whole foods contain the nutrients needed for digestion and all your bodily processes, refined foods do not. When you take in foods that are not whole your body has to withdraw nutrients from your cells, your savings account. This withdrawal process compensates for the refined foods' lack of nutritional value. Constantly withdrawing from your cells creates degenerative cells and eventually degenerative diseases. Remember the biology lesson above?

Back to the benefits of whole food eating, whole health living:

- healthy cells and all the rest of that biology stuff
- stable body weight, right where your weight should be for your height and frame size
- great energy all day long, no slumps and fuzzy periods so you can do all you enjoy doing and feel great
- good mood and positive mentality from healthy neuro-transmitters and hormone production

- good role model for your kids, friends, family -- the more people who eat whole foods, the better communities of vibrant, healthy, happy people we will have

- superb sleep because your body is not busy detoxing all kinds of refined food at night

- preventing and healing degenerative diseases while creating radiant and vibrant *whole health*!

Whole food eating and whole health living saves bundles of money that would be otherwise spent on prescription drugs, surgery, medical tests and treatments, chemo, and radiation. Does it not seem reasonable to put "an ounce" of money into good food and good living rather than "a pound" (more like a ton) of money into medical care for degenerative diseases?

The extra money spent on good food is your holistic health insurance, your preventative health plan. It is your way of preventing disease and all the decreased quality of life issues that go along with disease.

Please remember the seemingly cheaper cost of packaged foods is due to huge subsidies handed out to agri-business, large-scale farms getting huge tax

breaks and huge cash payments to raise monocrops of corn, soy, wheat, etc. These subsidized monocrops are then turned into hundreds of substances that go into packaged frankenfoods*. This is not healthy eating or living!

Methods of making Whole Food Eating Cost Efficient

Find your food from local farmers. Remove the long list of "middle men" between you and the food and the food will be cheaper. The

*frankenfoods — a term for foods that are so far removed from natural foods that they are scary to your body cells and your overall health!

farmer gets 100% of the profit and you get 100% of the local, whole food benefits.

Local food is fresher, seasonal and more nutritious. Fresh picked has 100% of the nutrition intact. Transporting fresh produce from thousands of miles away decreases the nutritional value quickly. Eating food that grows in season, in your local area, feeds your body better nutritionally and energetically. Our bodies thrive on food grown in the climate we actually live in.

See Chapter 4 for resources on locating local foods.

Learn to shop and prepare food wisely.

Buy in bulk: Dried beans are much cheaper than canned beans. Canned ones are handy in a pinch so keep a few cans on hand for quick meals.

Whole grains are cheaper than those ground into flour and in turn manufactured into bread, pasta, wraps, tortillas, etc. The more processes the whole food goes through before getting to your plate, the more it costs you to eat it. All whole grains can be cooked like brown rice. The cooking times will vary based upon the size of the whole grain.

Base your diet around cheaper, organically grown plant foods: such foods include vegetables, fruits, nuts, seeds, beans, and whole grains. Use animal products - meats, eggs, and dairy - in smaller servings.

Buying local meat, eggs and dairy directly from the farmer is a much cheaper option than at a supermarket: perhaps you may also want to learn to hunt and provide your own "wild" sourced meat! Once again you are not paying the middle men all their profits. The products are also far healthier. Make certain to ask your farmers how they raise their animals; are they feeding their animals grass and/or the actual natural foods that an animal would graze on if they were wild? OR are the animals being fed an unnatural diet of grains and foods they would not eat in the wild? Natural living makes for natural, balanced health.

Buy organic: fewer chemicals and better nutritional value. While organic foods seem to cost more than conventionally grown foods, the value of organics cannot be stressed enough. Foods grown organically, naturally, have higher nutritional values. Your body is in better nutritional health when you treat it naturally with whole foods and a whole health lifestyle. Plants and other animals react to natural foods and natural living in the same manner: their bodies are healthy and whole!

Think about biology, cell regeneration, your internal nutritional savings account; all are good reasons to put whole, organic nutrition into your body. You will save money by preventing disease while avoiding the need for health and medical intervention.

Environmental Working Groups list of 53 produce items from most to least contaminated: http://www.ewg.org/foodnews/list/ This can help you decide where to put your money if 100% organic produce is not possible.

Eat whole foods, not packaged foods, this includes packaged drinks. Drink water and make herb teas. Avoiding bottled water and other packaged drinks will save a bundle on the grocery bill as well as in your nutritional savings accounts. Let's examine soda: soda is high in sugar and carbonation that robs your savings account of minerals and nutrients. When you drink beverages that are not whole, you contribute to tooth decay, osteoporosis, cell degeneration, and disease. The beverage packages also contribute to our earth's garbage problem.

You ARE What You Eat!

This is a clichéd saying that drives people crazy! I hear responses all the time that go something like this, "do I look like broccoli, or carrots, or Twinkies for that matter?!"

This sort of logic is about the same as saying your house made of wood should look like a tree (now if you are an owl...). Does your house sprout leaves in the spring or showcase evergreen needles year round? Of course not!

You are what you eat is an expression of cell biology - human physiology at the basic level. Remember the cell biology talk above? Well, your body cells reproduce continually from the time you were conceived in your mom's fallopian tube until the day you gasp your last breath. Eat 100% whole foods and that last gasp will be much further in the future!

Your body cells can only be as healthy as the foods you put in your mouth. Food is the building block of your cells, of your whole body! Processed, refined foods make for processed and refined cells. Garbage in = garbage out. Whole foods make whole cells! Whole in = whole out!

Eat junk food, your body reproduces junk cells and slips and slides into degenerative health diseases.

Eat 100% whole foods, the only foods we had available to us prior to food manufacturers taking over the food scene, and you create 100% whole health cells. This creates a lifetime of vibrant, radiant, juicy good health for your cells, **your body**!

Moderation is the Key (when you are eating whole foods)

Whole food eating means eating like people did 200 years ago, before corporations took over our food scene. This means we need to eat the food we ate before we were inundated with packaged, processed, refined food products. The key word here is "products." They are not real food.

"Moderation is the key in everything we eat." I often hear people say this. I agree, if (and "if" is the operative word here), the foods are whole foods! Our bodies were not meant to eat refined foods. How can there be moderation in something that was never meant to be in our digestive tracts, our bodies, and disturbing our cellular health? I cannot stress this enough: eat for vibrant cellular health!

Moderation is not the key with "food products"! So what is the key? Simply this, elimination of refined foods from our lives! **Elimination** is **the key with refined foods!**

Here is my whole health mantra: Eat whole foods! Whole foods reproduce whole cells creating vibrant energy and lasting whole health!

Moderation *is* the key when eating whole foods.

This is a goal to work towards. **The more refined, packaged food you remove from your diet, the more quickly your body moves towards healing.** I am reminding you again that it is never too late, that there is hope for everyone to create healthy cells and a healthy body by moving to whole food eating. Refined foods damage our cells. If we eat 100% whole foods, healthy cell regeneration is 100%. Elimination of 100% of refined foods does wonders for your body cells, tissues, organs, organ systems, and the organism: **You!**

If "moderation" in regards to refined foods is the path you take, you will still be inflicting damage on body cells. I know this sounds harsh and you may be thinking "gosh, give us a break, Paula." The benefits of whole foods far outweigh the perceived pleasure of refined foods. Do your best and move in the direction of 100% whole food eating. Your whole health will thrive!

Self-Discipline vs. Self-Love, guilt is NOT part of the healing equation!*

"To enjoy good health, to bring true happiness to one's family, to bring peace to all, one must first discipline and control one's own mind. If

a man can control his mind they can find the way to Enlightenment,
and all wisdom and virtue will naturally come to him."

Buddha

Discipline of the mind is not will power. Will power is a fallacy. This fallacy creates only guilt. Health is not about guilt. it is about love - self-love! Love is all there is.

Love is the most powerful creative force in the universe. You are the result of what you love most.

You either love your health and feeling good in your body more than desserts and junk food, or you love desserts and junk food more. It is as simple as that. Don't beat yourself up thinking that you have no will power, no discipline. This only creates the guilt, binge, guilt, binge cycle that leaves us starving for more. More what? Certainly more food is not needed. Try loving yourself more.

Ask yourself this, what do you really love? One of the best ways to raise self-esteem is to make truly loving choices that lead to increased strength of body, mind, and soul. For example, if you truly love yourself when exercising, you then choose to walk or do whatever you do for exercise with a happy heart. At meal time and snack times, you pass on the refined foods and opt for nutrient dense, life giving whole foods. These are truly loving choices.

Self-love is real. Will power is a myth that only makes us feel guilty, frustrated, and give up on truly loving ourselves.

May your walk through life be about peace and love.

*This section was excerpted and then paraphrased, with permission, from a health article written by Michele Smith of Forever Fit with Michele, NYC

Chapter 3

50 Ways to Love Your Fruits and Vegetables!

"Eat food. Not too much. Mostly plants."

Michael Pollan

"I like fruits and vegetables... They are just healthy food. ....."

Student at GardenShare's Food Day Youth Summit 2011

I WOULD BE HORRIBLY REMISS if I did not include an inspirational Chapter on ways to increase the fruits and vegetables in your diet. These delicious and nutritious plant foods are powerhouses for our bodies' health, full of vitamins, minerals, enzymes, fiber, phytonutrients, anti-oxidants and a host of nutrients yet to be discovered. Eating fruits and vegetables helps to cleanse and rebuild our body right down to the cellular level. Yes, we are back at that cell biology issue again!

Suggestions for Loving Good Vegetables

I. Be adventurous, try new vegetables you have never cooked or tasted before. There are so many more than the tried and true potatoes, carrots, lettuce, broccoli (cucumbers, peppers, tomatoes are really fruit).

2. Find local farm stands, farm markets, and farmers who grow food sustainably. The food will be far more nutritious and you will be eating local, seasonal produce, not food shipped from thousands of miles away. Produce loses its nutritional value and vitality the longer it takes to travel to your plate.

3. Grow your own, even a small raised box or potted vegetables, to enjoy food fresh from the plant. Plant some berry bushes or maybe a fruit tree or two.

4. Make the commitment to eat at least 2 to 3 servings per meal and snack on vegetables and fruit when you need a between meal lift.

5. Make your plate mostly vegetables with high-quality, locally raised, grass-fed protein as the smaller portion on your plate. Add beans instead of the animal protein for another plant and fiber boost to your diet.

6. Add shredded carrots, beets, parsnips to your whole food baked goodies. A beet cake is a fun alternative to the well-loved carrot cake. See Chapter 10 for a taste tempting, whole food recipe.

7. Add beets, carrots, squash, and parsnips to pancakes and waffle batter. I even add spinach, kale, collards, etc. to my kids' pancakes. They used to call these "green" breakfast pancakes, *Shrek* pancakes, now they just label them as Mom's wacko healthy foods.

8. Make scrambled, poached or fried eggs, beans and greens for breakfast. Get your eggs locally from a farmer who lets the chickens feed naturally.

9. Make omelets with lots of vegetables, different than the typical ones put in omelets. Be creative and adventurous. Add fresh herbs!

10. Make a breakfast burrito with scrambled eggs (naturally raised ones, of course) and/or refried beans. Add plenty of vegetables and herbs and roll into a sprouted grain tortilla or a 100% whole grain tortilla, preferably organic so you can avoid genetically modified organisms, GMO's*. Also, try rolling the burrito fillings into large leaves of kale, collard, or Swiss chard and really up the veggie intake!

11. Make vegetable curries for dinner and use the leftovers for lunch or breakfast. Curried vegetables and beans, eggs, or meat are yummy for any meal. Think past the typical refined grain breakfasts that most Americans eat: processed cereals and milk, doughnuts and coffee, toast and juice. Start putting real food and vegetables into every meal.

12. Add hardy greens to soups, stews, stir fries: kale, collards, Swiss chard, dandelion greens, beet greens, spinach, arugula, mustard greens, endive, and escarole. Cut them into small, fine strips to make them more palatable to those persons new to eating greens.

13. Make fruit smoothies for breakfast or snacks. If you avoid dairy, see Chapter 10 for recipes on how to make fresh nut and seed milk. Making your own nut and seed milk avoids the packaged, processed, non-dairy milk. Remember to "chew" your smoothies. See Chapter 8 for more on chewing.

* GMOs are genetically modified organisms, in this case genetically modified foods. These are foods that have had their genetics manipulated in laboratories; they have had extra genes spliced into their genetic material. Examples are tomatoes with salmon genes spliced into them, supposedly to make the tomato more cold hardy. While this may make sense on some level to some people; did nature intend for tomatoes to have salmon genes? I think not. Me, I will go with nature's plan. She seems to know what she is doing!

14. Buy large carrots and make your own carrot sticks. Avoid packaged baby carrots. Most commercially packaged baby carrots are actually large carrots that were less than desirable (rotting), carved into baby carrot shapes and soaked in chemicals to kill microorganisms. This is not a healthy option.

15. Make "sticks" out of any root veggie that appeals to you, eat them plain, dip into hummus or other whole food spread or dip. Root vegetables: parsnips, celeriac, turnips, daikon radish, rutabaga, carrots, and beets. Dip recipes are in Chapter 10.

16. Snack on red pepper halves filled with hummus, yummy! Or fill them with fresh herbed cottage cheese. Use your imagination!

17. Make fruit salads with local, seasonal fruits.

18. Add new vegetables to your raw, green salads that you have never tried in a raw salad. Try anything!

19. Skip desserts and eat fresh, local, seasonal fruit. Off season? Try fruit you froze or canned or try organic frozen fruits.

20. Make homemade pizza with whole grain crust and load it up with vegetables. Eat with a salad greens and veggie salad or a shredded root veggie and cabbage salad. Have that fruit salad for dessert.

21. In the fall and winter, bake quantities of squash, sweet potatoes, or yams and keep the extra for quick meals and snacks.

22. Add extra squash and sweet potatoes to pancake and waffle batter.

23. Extra squash is also yummy added to "egg nog" smoothies. I even add cooked beets to get vegetables into my kids.

24. Avoid ready-to-eat packaged vegetables and fruits. Sure they are convenient but once produce is cut up it loses nutrients and starts to decompose faster. Most pre-cut fruits and vegetables are wet, an easy place for mold to grow.

25. Skip the "greens" in a salad and make a salad out of all kinds of raw chopped vegetables, grated root vegetables, and shredded cabbages. Mix it up and use simple oil and vinegar dressing.

26. Grill veggie chunks on kebabs.

27. Roast vegetables in the oven for fall and winter warming dishes. Try tourlou, a Greek roasted veggie delight! Recipe in Chapter 10.

28. Make big pots of soups and stews and eat all week. Think lots of vegetables.

29. At restaurants: skip the bread (it is refined flour anyhow) and ask for extra vegetables in your salad and as a side dish. Order pasta dishes without the pasta and have the chef put the pasta sauce on a pile of steamed vegetables instead. You avoid the refined flour pasta and get the benefits of vegetables. Skip any flour- based food when you are out and about (crackers, noodles, pasta, bread, desserts, white rice) and opt for extra vegetables instead.

30. Skip the factory-farmed meat at fast food restaurants (skip the fast food altogether, but if you find yourself with no other option...) eat a salad and baked potato with beans and salsa. Hopefully there is a salad bar with beans to add some digestive "staying" power to the vegetables. Protein and fat, balance out the meal, creating greater and longer satisfaction between meals.

31. Use whole grain quinoa, millet, amaranth, teff, or brown rice to make a "pasta" salad. You will be skipping the actual packaged pasta and using the whole grains instead. Then add far more vegetables to your whole grains than most people do to the average summertime pasta salads.

I will end here before I do hit 50 suggestions! Fruits are generally easy for people to add into their diet, vegetables are where people get stuck. Fruits and vegetables make for good cell replication - healthy cell biology! Remember: every step towards healthy, whole food eating creates positive changes in the health of your cells and your whole body. **There is hope and you are not too late!**

Chapter 4
Navigating Local / Seasonal Food

*"Live in each season as it passes; breathe the air, drink the drink,
taste the fruit, and resign yourself to the influences of each."*

Henry David Thoreau

"Local is the new organic."

Bill McKibben

Now THAT I HAVE CONVINCED you to eat lots of vegetables, (I have
convinced you, haven't I?)—Where do you find the best and most
nutritious produce?

Local food is out there! If you step out of the supermarket, away
from "corporate America" food, you will find a thriving community of
local growers just waiting to fill your table with healing, whole foods to
nourish and support you and your family's health.

Get in touch with the farmers who grow your food. Get in touch
with food; literally, touch it. Cut it up and prepare it yourself. When we
touch the food we prepare and eat, it helps to heal us.

**Choosing primarily local and seasonal foods is good for you, the
local economy, and the earth as a whole:**

You are getting food in its nutritional prime. It has not been hauled thousands of miles about the globe. This keeps the food's nutrients more intact so your cells thrive! Foods grown in local soil are attuned to the same climate and energy in which your body lives. Your cells recognize this and utilize everything more efficiently. An herbalist I trained under used to say this all the time: "Eat from under your own apple tree; eat from your own backyard!" It makes good health and healing sense!

Eating local keeps the farmer down the road, the next town over, or on the other side of the county working, and feeding their family. If we all concern ourselves with caring for our local economies, things would be better all over this Earth.

Local food helps the Earth as a whole. One simple way is the fuel oil that is saved by not moving food from Florida, California, Mexico, Guatemala, S. America, China, etc. Less fuel burned, less pollution, and all that the pollution brings to our environment.

Where to look for nutritious and delicious local foods:

Farmers Markets

Roadside farm stands: ask about the farmer's growing practice and their use of chemicals

CSA farms- Community Supported Agriculture, you buy a "food" subscription, investing in the farms production for the upcoming season and get fresh farm food weekly

Local food co-ops and health food stores

The farmer down the road - they may not have an actual farm stand but may be willing to share their harvest with you at a low cost.

Community gardens -- a fine option to grow food, find food, and connect with like-minded people.

Grow some in your own back yard! Share and swap food with a neighbor who grows food too!

To find local food, here are search resources:

http://www.localharvest.org/search.jsp

http://farmersmarket.com/search?utf8=%E2%9C%93andterm= 13676andas=location

http://search.ams.usda.gov/farmersmarkets/

Live in Northern NY? In and around St. Lawrence county:

www.gardenshare.org Try starting a similar non-profit in your community!

As websites may change, try a Google search for local food sources in your area: farm markets, CSA farms, etc. Use the web to search your local area for where great food is happening. You will find nourishing whole food and you may just make some amazing whole health friends!

Enjoy local food! It tastes better and nourishes your body and body cells better!

Chapter 5
Navigating the Whole Food Scene

"If you don't take care of your body, where are you going to live?"

Unknown

"The doctor of the future will no longer treat the human frame with drugs, but rather will cure and prevent disease with nutrition."

Thomas Edison

TRANSITIONING TO WHOLE FOOD EATING takes some creative re-thinking of how we do things in our world. We need to re-think how we function in our kitchens, how we stock our kitchens (which includes how we clean out the refined food from our non-whole food kitchens), how we shop, where we shop, and how we eat out with our best whole health in mind. Remember, the goal is to create vibrant cellular health which will have the ripple effect of vibrant human health!

Take Back Your Kitchen, Take Back Your Health

See this as an adventure, embarking on new territory in life to explore, experience, and incorporate health and healing into every cell! Have fun with it. See this as an opportunity for personal growth!

Our kitchens have been taken over by the corporate world, microwave ovens, takeout food and the resultant unhealthy foods from these spaces.

Human health requires real food, whole foods, to sustain cellular health, prevent degenerative diseases, and keep our bodies vibrantly healthy. Have I said this before?!

200 years ago, food did not come to us in the form of packaged, factory made "food products" or animal products from large, industrial "animal factories." Most peoples' food came from the backyard garden, barn yard, or another farmer down the way. People grew what they ate. They traded what they grew to acquire that which they did not grow.

This style of eating can be replicated closely enough through buying local food from farmers in your area. You then get the best of seasonal food, right when it is at the peak of freshness and nutritional value. Seek out farmers who care for their land, growing fields, and animals in a sustainable way. Look for organic and bio-dynamic methods of growing food. A farm does not have to be certified organic to be living and growing in sync with nature. I know many farmers in my area of northern NY State who are not organic certified but actually grow at standards way above federal organic standards.

This method of conscientious care of the land and all living things produces food with much higher nutritional values. And for the record, when produce has blemishes on it, it is a good thing. The blemishes mean the fruit or vegetable was defending itself against something. In this defense process, the plant makes many phyto-chemicals to fight the good vs. bad fight. Those phyto-chemicals are power nutrition for your cells! Perfect looking produce is an invention of agri-business. It is aesthetically pleasing, but seriously downgraded in nutritional value.

When your style of cooking and eating becomes 100% whole food utilizing lots of fresh, local and seasonal produce, your health will return

32

to the radiance nature intended. Humans sick with high blood pressure, high cholesterol, cardiovascular disease, obesity, diabetes, nervous system and immune system disorders (to name just a few) is not normal or natural. The body strives to be vibrantly healthy; nature meant us to be that way into our very old age. The advent of junk, fast, convenience, take out and manufactured foods is what is turning on our "sick" genes. This new style of eating is killing humans by the hundreds of thousands every year. And these deaths can be prevented.

Be brave. Stand up and refuse to eat "food products." Be a role model for your kids, your family, and your friends. Slowly but surely we can turn every kitchen back into a healing place, where food is our healing medicine and people take pride in what they prepare and share with the ones they love and feed. Really, is there any other way?

Kitchen Clean up

And no, I am not talking about washing dishes, mopping floors and cleaning the stove and counter tops.

Cleaning out your kitchen of "food products," anything that is not whole foods, is imperative to moving forward with healthy choices, whole food eating, and healing your body.

The easiest thing to do is remove all products that come in a box, bag, jar or can. Most of these "products" should never be called food. This simple cleaning act will get rid of everything you should re-learn to not eat. However, I will give more detail!

As you read on, there is a section on navigating the supermarket. I have given examples of foods that are packaged foods that are OK to keep in the kitchen. Not all of us are going to go back to making 100% of the foods we eat; nice idea but not terribly practical in today's world. Buying a jar of 100% natural, preferably organic, salsa is entirely different than buying a box of 'dinner' helper, a package of manufactured cookies, frozen dinners, or a frozen, and refined flour crust pizza.

Get rid of white flour and white sugar. This is the stuff sold in the five pound packages meant for baking treats that will kill your cellular health. Get rid of any products where white flour and white sugar appear as ingredients. White flour and white sugar are refined foods that rob your body of nutrition, are highly addictive, and create degenerative diseases in your body. Regular grocery store brown sugar is not any different. It is simply white sugar with added caramel coloring to make you think it is a healthier sugar. Trust me, it is **not!**

Get rid of all hydrogenated oils, partially hydrogenated oils, corn syrup, high fructose corn syrup and corn sugar (corn syrup's new name to make you think it is healthy). Get rid of vegetable oils. Most are cheap, highly refined and just plain bad for your health. Buy 100% extra virgin olive oil and use it very sparingly. It is pure fat, a concentrated food. Respect it. Butter, sesame oil and coconut oil are good for cooking.

I prefer butter; butter from pasture-raised, and grass-fed animals, that is. Butter is far more local, for me, than olive, sesame or coconut oil. I can make butter in my own kitchen from heavy cream from the cows down the road. On the other hand, I cannot grow coconuts, olives or sesame seeds.

Whole foods: this is your mantra, think whole foods. Get the stuff out of the kitchen that is not whole foods and stock your shelves with whole foods: raw nuts and seeds, dried beans, whole grains, fruits and vegetables, naturally raised animal products.

Toss out anything with artificial ingredients: preservatives, additives, coloring agents, emulsifiers, natural flavors (except real vanilla, most packaged foods use vanillin. It is fake.), artificial sweeteners, fake fats, etc. **Toss them out** of your food life. Your body cells and your life depend on it!

If this does not make sense, invite me over! HandsOnHealthHH. com I will go through the cupboards with you and help clean out the old and bring in the new: whole foods! I will also go with you to the supermarket and teach you how to shop for whole health, healing and lifetime vitality! Have fun cleaning out the kitchen, the "food products" and have a great day creating a healthier life!

Navigating the Whole Food Kitchen

A whole food kitchen is one that focuses on foods as they come from nature, not food from factories and manufactured, fake food-like substances. Processed cheese food product is an example of fake food. Just what is processed cheese food?!

You are about to embark on an amazing adventure of learning to gather and prepare real food from scratch! Your body will be nourished beyond your wildest idea of what good nutrition is and will shine with radiant health and high levels of energy.

You will have fresh, raw ingredients in your home. Foods you can eat in their raw state or prepare for consumption. You will no longer open boxes and bags of factory made foods to pop into the microwave and eat two and a half minutes later. Your food will burst with taste, texture and juiciness!

Whole food eating means eating like people did two hundred years ago, before corporations took over our food scene.

Keep your kitchen work simple.

Choose delicious and juicy food!

You are not giving up pleasure from food, your body WILL crave whole foods when your palate and taste buds detox from the harshness of refined salt, sugar, and packaged, refined foods. Your taste buds will burst with the flavor of real food, and your body will thank you with radiant health.

A whole food kitchen means stocking the refrigerator, shelves and cupboards with natural, fresh foods. See Chapter 2 for whole foods to stock in your new, vibrant health kitchen!

WHERE do I find whole foods? Health food stores, health food sections of supermarkets, local food co-ops, the outer sections of super-markets (the inner aisle tend to be where the crappy packaged foods are), road side farm stands, CSA farm shares, farmers' markets, your local farmer down the road that you haven't yet met. Remember to ask how they raise their produce and animals. Insist on the best for your body and your family's bodies!

WARNING! In twenty years of doing whole food education with individuals, I see this challenge over and over: Just because a food is sold in a health food store, perhaps is also labeled "organic," does not mean it is a healthy food for your body. Food manufacturers of "healthy foods" also realize there is money to be made on packaged snack and junk foods. While organic potato chips are much healthier than their main stream counter-parts, they are still potato chips... Not a health or life-giving food. This goes for organic cookies and treats, gluten-free products, other snacks and goodies. They are not healthy just because they are sold in a health food store. **Think whole foods in every purchase you make. Learn to check the ingredients. Do not rely on the "health claim" on the front of the package.** Always ask yourself: "How far is this food from how nature made it?"

Navigating Food Labels

Food labels are easy to read and understand; it is simply a matter of practice and familiarizing yourself with labels. Obviously, the easiest and best food choices are 100% whole foods, no label reading needed! Whole apples, carrots, broccoli, kale, onions, etc. do not need labels. No human interference has occurred to add synthetic ingredients or remove healthy nutrients, as long as they are organically grown and non-GMO. We will not get into the various Frankenfoods here!

"If people let the government decide what foods they eat and what medicines they take, their bodies will soon be in as a sorry state as the souls who live under tyranny."

Thomas Jefferson

Learning to navigate a supermarket that is chock full of extremely unhealthy *food products* will truly save your life! The first place you want to look is on the list of ingredients. Every ingredient listed on the label should be 100% natural, whole foods. The ingredient list should be short, 5-8 whole foods. Longer ingredient lists are usually a very clear indication of "too much synthetic" in the product. Sound advice for long ingredient lists: Put the product back and step away from the shelves! Your health and life depend on it!

IGNORE health claims on labels. Health claims are a marketing ploy that serves at least 3 purposes:

1.   Leads you to believe it is healthy so that you buy, buy, buy the product.

2.   Diverts your attention from where it truly needs to be, the ingredient list.

3.   To make you believe that this is THE food that is going to save you from food hell and damnation.

It is all BS! Just read the ingredients, please. An example of this strategy in action is "gluten-free" packaged foods. I have clients tell me all the time that they buy gluten-free products because they think they are healthy. "Gluten-free must be healthy, the products are made for people with celiac disease," is the logical explanation I hear.

There are filler ingredients in gluten-free products. Some of these fillers are potato starch, white rice flour, corn and tapioca starch... these refined ingredients are setting you up for blood sugar and insulin issues which leads to diabetes! Buy whole food, gluten-free products or learn to make your own.

I will insert two ingredient lists for gluten-free bread. Read and think about which one seems whole and natural. Use this thought process to make decisions on what food choices will nourish your body and what food choices will deplete your nutritional stores, your nutritional savings account.

White Rice Loaf: Ingredients: Filtered water, rice flour, tapioca starch, high oleic safflower oil, pear juice concentrate, yeast, organic tapioca syrup, methylcellulose, orange citrus fiber, salt, sodium carboxymethylcellulose, calcium phosphate, glucono delta lactone. Enriched with thiamin, riboflavin, niacin, iron and folic acid.

Brown Rice Loaf: Ingredients, all organic: brown rice flour, deep well water, brown rice, ground flax seeds, unrefined olive oil, rice sourdough culture, unrefined sea salt, (may contain traces of sesame seeds).

Both of these rice loaf ingredient lists are "gluten-free." Which one would you choose as part of a whole food diet?

Think about this: Two hundred years ago no one had to read labels and the health claims on food labels. Why? Because food labels basically did not exist. People ate what grew locally, from their back yard, and what was available seasonally. Mass production of manufactured food did not begin until late in the nineteenth century.

Completely avoid:

1. All sugars and sweeteners, including and especially artificial ones. Holiday celebrations are okay but remember that every day is not a holiday. Learn to bake and enjoy whole food treats for holidays, birthdays, and any celebratory events.

2. Hydrogenated oils and partially hydrogenated oils; these are nasty trans-fats.

3. Corn syrup, high fructose corn syrup, corn sugar, fructose.

4. Chemicals or any ingredient you cannot pronounce.

5. Artificial food colorings.

6. Artificial flavorings. If it has to be flavored, seriously, it must be gross!

7. Preservatives, MSG, BHA, BHT, Nitrates and Nitrites.

8. Nutrients added to fortify or enrich. Synthetic nutrients are added to *food products* otherwise they have zero nutritional value.

9. Fillers and texture enhancers.

10. Artificial colors.

11. Cheap vegetable oils: soy, canola, and corn are examples. Experts may recommend canola, I avoid it. It is highly GMO and suspect as a healthy food, in my opinion. Do your own research, form your own opinion. I prefer to stick to traditional foods that have been used over the centuries!

12. Refined flours: white, unbleached, all-purpose, cake, any and all flour that is not 100% whole grain.

If an ingredient name on the label looks un-natural it more than likely is un-natural. Assume it is. In this instance, assuming can save your life!

Below are the ingredients lists from two top, brand name food manufacturer's products. The pasta sauce ingredients look reasonable, whole, and nutritious. In the second list of ingredients I have bold faced those ingredients that I would not put in my body. My reasons for avoiding these ingredients: they are not whole foods, they are from questionable origins, and they are genetically modified ingredients. This is the process I use to evaluate the ingredients in packaged foods, to decide if I want to put them in my body and have those ingredients influencing the replication of my body cells.

Pasta Sauce Ingredients: (all organic) tomatoes in juice, tomato puree, naturally milled sugar, sweet basil, sea salt, extra virgin olive oil, garlic, natural calcium chloride, black pepper fennel, oregano. *I would prefer a sauce without added sugar but this is next to impossible to find.*

An Easy Meal "Manufactured, Packaged" **Sauce Ingredients:** Water, **Canola Oil, Roasted Corn,** Cheese Paste (Monterey Jack Cheese [Milk Cultures, Salt, Enzymes], Cheddar Cheese [Milk Cultures, Salt, Enzymes], Surface Ripened Semisoft Cheese [Milk Cultures, Salt, Enzymes], Whey, Water, Salt),**Modified Food Starch,** Jalapeno Peppers, Diced Tomatoes in Tomato Juice, Red Peppers, Cooked Black Beans, **Dehydrated Cream** (Cream [Milk], Nonfat Milk, Soy Lecithin), Contains Less than 2% of: Salt, Cream (Milk), **Sugar,** Roasted Red Peppers, Vegetables (Onions, Carrots, Celery), Dehydrated Chili and Chipotle Peppers, **Soy Protein Concentrate,** Dehydrated Onions, **Spice,** Olive Oil, **Flavoring,** Molasses, **Yeast Extract,** Lime Juice Concentrate, Garlic, Vinegar, Dehydrated Garlic, **Natural Smoke Flavoring.**

More Label Tips

Learn about the sugars in manufactured foods. Any ingredient that ends in "ose" is a form of sugar. Corn syrup and high fructose corn syrup are also forms of sugar. Fruit juice sweetened products are still sweetened with sugar, perhaps a better option that corn syrup, but sugar none the less.

Learn to read labels for sugar information and content. 4 grams of sugar equals 1 teaspoon of sugar. If a serving of a product has 24 grams of sugar, there are 6 teaspoons of sugar per serving of this product. That is a hefty dose of sugar.

As an example, let's look at plain yogurt. Plain yogurt is heated milk that has cultures added to the milk to make it ferment into yogurt. A six ounce serving of plain yogurt has 9 grams of sugar. This is 100% milk lactose, which is natural milk sugars. Now add flavorings and sweeteners to that plain yogurt and you can have 20, 30 or more grams of sugar in a 6 ounce serving.

Let's pretend we have a 6 ounce flavored yogurt that contains 24 grams of sugar. Now we will grab an empty ¾ measuring cup (which is 6 ounces) and add 6 teaspoons of sugar. This is the typical amount of added sugar in flavored yogurts. Six ounces equals 36 teaspoons; six out of thirty teaspoons six are pure sugar. A lesson to learn from reading yogurt labels is to buy plain yogurt, preferably from grass-fed and naturally raised animals. Add your own fruit, vanilla, cinnamon, and a tiny amount of sweetener, preferably not refined, white sugar!

Ask yourself these questions: Are there trans-fats in the product? What is the protein content of the product? Learn your food sources of fats, proteins and whole, complex carbohydrates. This knowledge will help you read and understand food labels better.

Take a deep breath and make good 100% whole food choices and feel your body reap the health benefits. The choice to be healthy takes time, conscious thought about your choices, and using good common sense. Eventually, the process becomes ingrained, second nature!

(See the quote at the beginning of Chapter 7)

Navigating the Supermarket for:
Whole Food Shopping, Cooking and Eating

Eating the whole food way takes conscious thought. Eventually it does become second nature. It is truly a process of retraining your thoughts, choices, and taste buds and using good 'ol common sense. Once you start and truly dedicate your choices to whole foods you will be amazed at how vibrant you feel and how natural and yummy real food tastes.

I am constantly asked questions like: "how do you do it, eat whole foods all the time, when there are so many packaged food choices right in front of us all the time?" My answer is simple. Two hundreds years ago these packaged foods would not have been available. Therefore, they are not real food in my eyes. Things that are not real foods are just not a choice to eat. Nature did not intend them to be put in our bodies. Our cells, genes, and chromosomes do not know what to do with them. The synthetic substances and combinations of substances in packages foods actually turn on our genes in negative ways, towards disease and death. These substances also make manufactured foods very addicting, like drugs to our bodies. Making the choice to not eat these substances was quite simple for me. I just remind myself that they were never a choice before the manufacturing of factory foods.

When you look at a food item, ask yourself: Did this come from nature? Was it manufactured? Nature Rules! Go with nature to feel your vibrant best health way into your very old age!

How to Shop

Shop for food asking yourself the "nature vs. manufactured" food question. This simple question makes choosing healthy foods easy!

Shop the perimeter of the supermarket: fresh fruits and vegetables, meats, eggs, milk and dairy products. Opt for choices that were naturally grown and raised. Buy the very best food your budget can afford. Team up with local farmers and producers and buy cheaper when you buy directly from the food source!

Avoid the supermarket bakery section. It is 100% processed, refined flours and sugars, and tons of synthetic additives that will make your body sick. Buy whole grain breads from a reputable bakery. Most of the packaged breads in the supermarket are of poor quality also. Read labels! If the bread is 100% whole grains without hydrogenated oils, corn syrup or corn sugar, unhealthy vegetable oils like canola, corn or soy, and synthetic ingredients, then it is an okay choice. Truthfully, such products are few and far between. Reading labels becomes highly important, anything that does not look like a nature-made ingredient probably is not. It is in your best interest to avoid these "bread" packaged foods.

Making your own whole grain bread and flour products can be a wonderful option. I make whole grain breads, pitas, bagels, muffins, cookies, cakes, pie crusts (I think you get the picture!) with 100% whole grain flours. I replace every ingredient in a recipe with a whole food substitute and create nutritious and delicious foods.

If you do not have the time or interest to bake, a great place to get quality breads is Little Stream Bakery in Canada if you live in the North Eastern United States, close to Canada. (www.littlestream.com) There are many whole grain bakeries across the United State. Search them out. It is well worth your time and effort to have good whole grains breads. Try typing "whole grain bakers cooperative" into a Google search.

Avoid the center of the supermarket, where all the packaged products live on shelves. Here you will experience huge quantities of factory made *food products*. Please do not mistake them for real food; they are not!

The center of the supermarket does have *some* redeeming products. I suggest you learn to shop with consciousness to what the label tells you about ingredients. If you could have made the product at home with fresh, whole food ingredients, the packaged version can be a healthy, time saving alternative in your whole food kitchen. Look for labels with very few and all-natural ingredients. If you cannot pronounce it and you have no idea if it was actually grown in nature, put it back on the shelf and walk away with your cellular health intact!

Examples of food products **that can be whole and natural:**

Salsa: are all ingredients in the salsa fresh fruits and vegetables, herbs and spices? Is the salsa free from sweeteners, preservatives, chemical sounding ingredients you cannot buy in the produce section? Avoid salt enhanced products unless it is unrefined sea salt that is used.

Pasta sauces: use the same logical questions as for the salsa.

Canned organic tomatoes and tomato paste: for making your own pasta sauces, soups, and stews. These products would be best purchased in glass jars or cans that are not lined in plastic. Tomato products are acid and leach toxins from the plastics.

So much to think about when moving through those aisles!

Canned organic beans: (chick peas, black beans, kidney beans, etc.) useful to have on hand when soaking and cooking dried beans is just not an option. Look for sea salt on the label not refined table salt.

Tortilla chips: made from organic, whole corn with no synthetic ingredients. Organic corn is not GMO*, genetically modified.

Granola cereals: look for brands that are not loaded with sugar and synthetic ingredients. Also, avoid the soy, canola and corn oils that are cheap, unhealthy, and used in some lesser quality granola.

Organic dark chocolate: a great replacement for commercial chocolate bars. You will love it and it is loaded with anti-oxidants! The commercial chocolates will have a plastic aftertaste when you finally make the switch to organic and fair-trade! Remember to savor it, small bits at a time, not a whole chocolate bar in one sitting! I am not trying to trade off sugar addictions for a *healthier* sugar addiction. My advice is to use organic chocolate as a treat. An even better lifestyle choice would be to get addicted to apples, carrots, beets, squash, pears, peaches, kale, collards...

*Genetically modified foods are another "frankenfood" nightmare. How did we, as a human culture, get to this crazy point? My answer: basic human greed. Natural foods cannot be patented and profited from, GMO and factory made foods can!

I hope this helps you to navigate the supermarket making whole food choices to enhance your health and the health of the planet.

Making Any Recipe a Whole Food recipe

Recipes from any cookbook can be converted into a whole food recipe: entrees, breads, desserts and treats, salads and dressings, sauces, soups, stews, anything! The trick is very simple: read the recipe and think about each ingredient in a whole food version. Just replace everything with whole foods!

Cooking fruits and vegetables: most recipe cooking times create over-cooked fruits and vegetables. Cook fruits and vegetables so they have some crispness or until they are just softening. You want to keep some snappy crispness and color. Brightly colored raw produce should still be brightly colored after you have gently cooked it.

Replace any refined flour with 100% whole grain flour. An approximate conversion is I cup refined flour = ¾ cup whole grain flour. Learn to play with your recipes to get the right consistency for whatever you are making or baking. Cake or muffin batter is obviously more fluid in consistency than cookie or bread dough.

Replace refined sugar with Rapadura, Sucanat sugar or maple syrup. If the recipe calls for 2 cups of sugar, immediately decrease it to I cup or less of the Rapadura or Sucanat. Truthfully, I would use one-half to two-thirds a cup of Rapadura sugar for a recipe that calls for 2 cups of refined sugar. This decreases the sweetness of the food, lowers the calories and makes it healthier for your body.

If you are using Maple Syrup as the sweetener, reduce the syrup by one-half. The syrup is much sweeter. I may even cut the amount of syrup to one-quarter to one-half cup of maple syrup to replace the original two cups of refined sugar the recipe calls for. This makes the recipe less sweet and better for you. You will get used to and appreciate cakes, cookies, brownies, muffins, pies, etc. that are less sweet. You will feel better with less blood sugar swings and the resultant sugar hangovers!

For recipes you are not cooking: raw, local honey is a good sweetener. one cup of honey is equal to two cups of white sugar. I would then cut the amount in half and use only one-quarter to one-half cup honey.

Replace fruits and vegetables in recipes with fresh, locally, and organically grown fruits and vegetables instead of frozen and canned.

Replace meat, eggs, and dairy with fresh, local, pasture-raised, grass or naturally fed equivalents.

Replace beans with organically grown beans you soak and cook yourself. Keep canned organic beans handy to use in a pinch. We all need easy steps from time to time!

Replace nuts and seeds with organic, raw options. Except for peanuts, always use roasted peanuts. Peanuts are actually legumes, beans, not nuts. They are prone to mold growth and are best roasted.

Use grass-fed, pasture-raised plain yogurt instead of sour cream. I have yet to find a good quality sour cream. The plain yogurt from grass-fed, pasture-raised animals will have a good fat/protein balance and healthy fats from being grass-fed and pasture-raised. You could make your own sour cream using pasture-raised, grass-fed heavy cream and cultures.

Yogurt can be used to make all kinds of creamy salad dressings and sauces. My best advice is to look at the spice and whole food ingredients on a commercial salad dressing label and replicate the flavor with yogurt and the same spices. This avoids the chemicals, cheap vegetable oils, and artificial ingredients in commercial products.

Replace vegetable oils with cold-pressed extra virgin olive oil for raw use in salad dressings, and on bread, pasta, and vegetables. Unrefined, sesame oil is great for stove top cooking. I prefer grass-fed, pasture-raised butter in both my stove top cooking and my baking (get rid of any hydrogenated vegetable oil shortenings and products, they will kill you!).

I oven roast vegetables in a 50-50 olive oil and butter blend at 325 degrees. (Higher heat burns butter and oils.) I also prefer that same grass-fed butter on bread, toast, pasta and vegetables. A fresh herbed butter pesto is divine on all these foods as well.

Get rid of any recipe ingredient that is fake food. Fake food kills body cells and ultimately will kill you. I want you to be healthy and love good, whole food!

Navigating Eating Away from the Whole Food Kitchen: Learning to Eat WHOLE On the GO!

Over the years, I have learned to be prepared and always take food with me. This is great for work and day trips. For longer stays away from home and when taking food with you is not an easy option, learning to navigate food choices when you eat out is quite simple.

The first step is simply thinking whole food, whole health. Use the same logic used when navigating the supermarket: ask yourself how close is the food in question to natural, whole, and real?

Avoid fast food restaurants (watch the movie *Supersize Me* if in doubt). High-quality, nutritious food is not on fast food restaurants radar. It is all about ingredients that are as cheap as possible and sold at the highest profits possible. Profit before people is the name of this game!

Remember, you are the customer in restaurants. Pleasing you should be the intention of the staff and owner. I often take ingredients I see on the menu and re-configure them into meals of my own creation.

Center your choices around nicely prepared vegetable dishes with protein sides: meat, eggs, and beans.

So a meal may be salad, chicken, or another meat option, and extra vegetables. The general vegetable serving that comes with meals is small because most people do not eat them! Ask for extra vegetables!

Examples: I generally do not eat bread, pasta, noodles, tortillas etc. when out in restaurants. They are always made from processed, refined flour, unlike the 100% whole grain choices I have at home.

At Mexican restaurants I ask for the corn tortillas instead of flour tortillas. Flour tortillas are refined flour. Ask for corn tortillas when you are ordering the fajitas that you put together at the table or you are ordering burritos. I have even taken my 100% sprouted whole grain tortillas with me, order the fajita fixings and used my own whole food tortilla. Other times I order the bowl of black beans or black bean soup and a large order of guacamole and skip flour products all together.

Instead of pasta, I order a pile of steamed vegetables with the pasta sauce over the vegetables. No pasta needed!

Skip the bread brought out at the beginning of the meal. It is 100% refined white flour, basically baked loaves of wall-paper paste. This refined flour bread *will* "glue up" your intestinal tract contributing to many digestive tract disorders and health problems.

Order burgers without the bread unless the restaurant has a 100% whole grain option. The secret is to look at the sandwich menu. Whole grain may not be offered with the burger section of the menu **but** there are whole grain breads available for the sandwiches made in the restaurant. Just ask for the whole grain sandwich bread with your burger. The more people ask for 100% whole grain options, the sooner restaurants will start serving them!

For lunches out, order a sandwich on whole grain bread. Unless the restaurant is very conscious of real food, most of the whole grain bread offered is only partially whole grain. Truly the bread is generally made with very little whole grain. Most often, restaurant whole grain bread is merely a loaf of supermarket wheat bread that is far less then whole or healthy. OR…

Opt for a salad with healthy greens (not iceberg lettuce) and lots of fresh vegetables. Go easy on dressings as they have nasty synthetic ingredients in them, opt for olive oil and vinegar or bring your own olive oil, apple cider vinegar, and herb dressing to the restaurant with you. Yes, I do this! I have learned to be prepared to keep synthetic ingredients and unhealthy vegetable oils out of my meals. All commercially prepared salad dressings are soy, canola, and/or corn oil which are all unhealthy options.

When eating breakfast out you can opt for poached eggs, omelets with vegetables and real cheese (not the American, sliced, processed cheese food. Whatever that is!), and ask for whole grain toast or go without toast and ask for extra vegetables. Get a bowl of oatmeal and skip the sugar. Get some fruit instead. The sugar will be refined white sugar and most restaurants do not have real maple syrup. Ask for some cinnamon to add to your oatmeal or carry a small container with you. I also carry a small container of real vanilla extract.

Skip the pancakes, French toast, and waffle options unless the restaurant has 100% whole grain options. This, as stated above, is a very rare find! Some places will have whole grain bread for sandwiches, again probably not 100% whole grain, but they are generally willing to make your French toast with this.

Be a menu detective and look at all the options! Be assertive and ask questions. Always remember, you are the customer and the owners **do** want you to be happy and come back. It is your health that is at stake, so ask questions and opt for whole foods!

Skip desserts in restaurants. They are the pit of white flour, white sugar, hydrogenated oils, corn syrups and corn sugar, cheap and unhealthy vegetable oils (soy, corn, canola) and other synthetic ingredients. Need I say more?

Learn to make desserts at home from whole food ingredients. Learn to enjoy desserts at home where you have control of the life and health giving ingredients.

The more people who ask about and insist on healthy choices while eating out, the more restaurants will rise to the occasion and start serving whole, fresh, real food!

When you no longer live and feel this *processed food* lifestyle, it is very noticeable when you do have a refined food day. The after affects linger for a day or two. This is called a *food hangover**!

I want health and whole real food to be easy and fun for you. When your body adjusts to real food, there is no going back! Manufactured foods are plastic tasting to your taste buds. They have bad after tastes too and the *food hangover* * from toxic synthetic ingredients is very apparent.

The sad thing is that most Americans feel this way every day of their lives from their refined, processed, packaged food diets: low level energy, hazy head, gut disturbances, bloated, the energy slump in the mid-afternoon, poor sleep quality (the body is struggling to detox the processed synthetics out of your body at night), mood swings, cravings for more of the refined foods, depression and anxiety from poor nutrition, PMS, acne and skin disturbances, reproductive tract issues. The list is never ending.

Are you convinced that whole foods are the way to live and create vibrant, whole health? This is my hope for you!

Eat Healthy, Eat Whole Foods!

*Food hangover is the ill feeling your body experiences after ingesting food products that are less than whole and/or are full of synthetic substances. This feeling can happen almost immediately after eating the food product and/or can last for days.

Chapter 6
Navigating Fitness

Yes, Exercise! Playful, Fun Exercise!

"Walking is man's best medicine."

Hippocrates

"Those who think they have no time for exercise will sooner or later have to find time for illness."

Edward Stanley

WHAT SELF-RESPECTING HEALTH PROMOTION PROFESSIONAL would not write about exercise? The human body was made to move. It is poetry in motion from a physiological, anatomical, and literal sense. Go ahead, get out there and move! Body movement is beautiful!

Why Exercise? There *are* good reasons, right?

Exercise, coupled with whole food eating and a whole health lifestyle, will keep you young. That is correct. This is your chance at slowing the aging process, your personal fountain of youth. Exercise is a powerhouse that keeps your muscles, nervous system, ALL internal organs and bones strong and dynamic. Every cell in your body benefits from the movement! Cell biology, baby, cell biology!

Just getting outside for thirty minutes of walking every day is a body bonus. I advise my clients to get on the floor and do a few push-ups and abdominal exercises, walk thirty minutes (or more if time and your heart and soul are into it, think of it as meditation in motion! More on that in the next Chapter.), and repeat the push-ups and abdominal work when you get back from your glorious, soul-soothing walk.

This is exercise that is simple, and no equipment required but a comfortable pair of shoes. Personally, I walk in Teva sandals or an inexpensive pair of soft soled water shoes, the kind that stretch and slip on. Water shoes are very comfy and grip the ground! Of course, the winters in Northern NY State requires a bit more foot coverage!

The benefits of exercise seem to be getting more media attention. I am completely amazed that this is not common sense! We need research to prove that moving our body, the way nature intended, is good for us? What has happened to our human collective common sense?

Ok.... let's look at the benefits of daily exercise:

Keeps you young. Workouts such as brisk walking or cycling boost the amount of oxygen consumed during exercise. Improving your aerobic capacity by just fifteen to twently percent would be like shaving ten to twenty years off your age. Every minute of good exercise, and it does not need to be hard, pounding exercise, adds two to three minutes to your life! Can you get payoffs like that with any other investment? Aerobic exercise may also stimulate the growth of new brain cells in older adults. Makes sense to me that it stimulates the growth of new brain cells in anyone who exercises!

Reduces infections. Moderate workouts temporarily rev-up the immune system by increasing the aggressiveness or capacity of immune cells. That may explain why people who exercise catch fewer colds.

Prevents heart attacks. Not only does exercise raise "good" HDL cholesterol and lower blood pressure, but new research shows it reduces arterial inflammation, another risk factor for heart attacks and strokes.

Eases asthma. New evidence shows that upper-body and breathing exercises can reduce the need to use an inhaler in mild cases of asthma.

Controls blood sugar. Exercise helps maintain a healthy blood-sugar level by increasing the cells' sensitivity to insulin and by controlling weight. Regular brisk walking can significantly cut the risk of developing type 2 diabetes.

Protects against cancer. Exercise may reduce the risk of colon-cancer by speeding waste through the gut and lowering your insulin level and blood sugar levels. It may also protect against breast and prostate cancer by regulating hormone levels.

Combats stress. Regular aerobic exercise lowers levels of stress hormones. For many people, exercise helps relieve depression as effectively as antidepressant medication.

Better sleep. A body that moves daily will sleep better for all reasons: physical, mental, emotional, and spiritual. Make it outdoor exercise and the fresh air and natural light exposure increases this benefit many times over!

Prevents and restores bone loss. Moving your body keeps the bones healthy and young. The bone cells lay down more new bone, preventing and reversing osteoporosis.

Stronger muscles, better flexibility and balance. Exercise keeps your muscles strong. Moving through full range of motion everyday keeps your muscles, tendons, ligaments, and joints flexible and strong. Exercise creates balance in body, mind, and spirit. Yoga is one great way to increase your muscle strength while creating better flexibility and balance for ease of movement!

Better organ function and health. Anything that makes your body stronger is going to make all organs, right down to your very cells, function better. Better circulation means better oxygen and nutrition being transported to the cells and better waste removal from the cells. This makes for healthier cells, organs and ultimately a healthier *You!*

Protect female and male health. Full body exercise keeps your sex hormones balanced: this means goodbye PMS and menopausal symptoms, hello healthy life! Increasing fitness by walking or practicing yoga enhances mood and reduces some menopausal symptoms, such as hot flashes and night sweats. Men benefit with lower incidence of erectile problems and increased overall "male" healthiness. Pelvic exercises, called kegel exercises, help prevent reproductive and urinary organ prolapse, clitoral erectile dysfunction and urinary leaking in females; erectile dysfunction and possibly benign prostate enlargement, a common cause of urinary problems in males. Women benefit as they have the same erectile tissues in their external genitalia. Men, despite not having a monthly menstrual flow, do have a monthly hormonal cycle. Regular exercise keeps this sex hormone cycle at top notch function. Because all body hormones and chemicals work in synergy, healthy sex hormones keep the rest of your body chemistry humming along in great health. Got those walking shoes on your feet? Heading out the door?

Weight loss and loss of belly fat. We are back to the common sense thing again, moving your body, as opposed to sitting on the couch, will keep you naturally thinner. The body was meant for movement, so it stands to reason it will be thinner with less belly fat than an inert body mass! Forty-five minutes of moderate-to-vigorous exercise in the morning may actually reduce your food cravings so you eat less all day. That is a healthy body bonus!

Reduces Inflammation. Inflammation in the body is the precursor to chronic lifestyle diseases. Reduce your bodily inflammation, and you reduce disease.

Regulates your appetite, reduces cravings, promote healthy digestion. When you feel good from moving, you are more apt to want to accentuate these good feelings with good food, avoiding the junk. When you eat good food and feel great, you are more apt to feel like moving. What a wonderful catch 22!

Lowers LDL cholesterol and triglycerides, raises HDL cholesterol. Trust me, you want this to happen!

Improve mood, concentration, nervous system function, and memory. Healthier bodies with healthier circulation means healthier brains for both intellectual and mood functioning!

Genetics. Your body will express its positive, healthy genes (epigenetics) when you exercise and eat 100% whole foods. Whole Health lifestyles turn off the negative genes that cause disease. Start flicking those healthy genes switches on today; *Get Moving!*

Attraction. Exercising makes us more attractive to others in mind, body and soul. We will attract to us people who have similar healthy lifestyles.

Prolong life. I think we are back to number one: exercise keeps you young! Studies lasting many years have consistently shown that being active cuts the risk of premature death by about 50 percent for men and women. You have mitochondria in your body cells; these are the powerhouses of the cells. When you exercise, you produce more and healthier mitochondria. This means your body functions better energetically, your metabolism is higher, and you live longer because of your powerful powerhouses!

FUN! Exercise increases the fun factor in your life. Do things that make you happy. If running is not your thing, do not do it just because it is supposedly "healthy." Do whatever makes your heart sing. Find several options that make you happy to move and mix them up. Every day do something that makes you feel good inside and out! This is your dose of daily fun that keeps you happy all day and night. Remember the sleep and lower stress benefits of exercise?

Exercise with a friend or a group of friends and create community. Healthy friendships up the fun factor of exercise and give you a positive support group from which to draw strength.

How to Exercise

As a physical education teacher, I was trained to think in the specifics of exercise: how much to do, for how long, at what intensity, and how often.

This is what I think about this manner of prescribing exercise: for most people it is too complicated and turns it into an intellectual process when, exercise is inherently a physical process. People tend to give up when they have to think too much about doing every step of the process correctly.

I will not give you specifics such as: you need to warm up at forty to fifty percent of your heart rate max for five to ten minutes, then work out at eighty percent of heart rate max for a minimum of thirty minutes and now cool down at forty to fifty percent of heart rate max for another five to ten minutes followed by a real slow down to normal movement intensity. Really? Who wants to spend all this time on these specifics? It gets confusing for most people. The inclination is to throw up one's hands in despair and frustration opting to sit in front of the TV or computer instead.

My fitness prescription is to find something you like to do and do it, preferably every day. Shake it up; have a few things you like to do and do something different every other day or so. I cannot express the value of a brisk paced walk every day, preceded and followed by core body-abdominal exercises and upper body-strength work. This can be as easy as some crunches and a few push-ups. Simple, easy to do and no equipment needed. You are working towards fitness without having to over-think the whole process with times, heart rates, and "routines" that supposedly create the best level of fitness!

Let's go back two hundred years again and think with our common sense. Did people concern themselves with how to best exercise for full body fitness? No, they just moved every day because their life circumstances included movement in everything they had to do to survive.

"We have witnessed the transformation of a world where calories were scarce and hard to get and physical activity was unavoidable into a world where physical activity is scarce and hard to get and calories are unavoidable."
[Any wonder why we have an obesity epidemic?! (My words.)]

David Katz, MD

Bottom Line

Create a space in your life so that exercise becomes a part of who you are. If labeling something as exercise makes you cringe and not want to do it, then call it "walking the dog." Dogs need to get out and have movement, fresh air, and natural light just like all humans do. No dog? How about borrowing the neighbor's dog for a walk? Ask the neighbor to go along with you and their dog for companionship and creating community!

You brush your teeth every day because this practice is good for your oral health. You create a space for teeth brushing to happen because it is good for you and for your health. Movement is also. Create the space for movement in your life and move!

Think about how you can make this an easy habit to follow through on: a creation of movement! If getting to the gym or an exercise class means twenty minutes of preparation before you even leave your house, twenty minutes of driving to the gym or class space, an hour of class time and then reversing the twenty minute drive and twenty minute preparation time (now cleanup and putting away equipment); you have just spent over 2 hours for 1 hour of movement. So many people state that lack of exercise is due to their time constraints. Go out for a brisk 30-40 minute walk, do some push-ups and core body strengthening movements, and call it a day. **Time saved:** over 1 hour *and* the dog walked! Dogs need exercise too!

Simply Put

Just do something **and do it every day!**

Motivate the mind; the body will follow.

Exercise is part of a Whole Health Lifestyle. Couple it with whole food nutrition and other whole health lifestyle choices, and this winning combination cannot be beat. It truly is a symphony of events, all of your whole health choices working in synergy with one another. It is nature's plan for all of us.

Need I say more? Are you convinced? Please, keep in mind that over-doing exercise, seriously pounding the body from high intensity training is not the same as regular daily exercise. Intense training may actually age the body faster.

Excess physical exercise is a stress on the body. Physical, emotional, or spiritual stress is negative for your health and creates a physiological response encouraging your body to hold onto fat.

Get outside. Move. You get the added benefit of fresh air and natural light. Your body will thank you in ways you can only imagine so let your imagination run wild (or walk wild)!

P.S. Just a word from Garfield... "I think that tossing and turning all night should be counted as exercise!"

Chapter 7
Exercising Your Mind, Body, and Soul Connection

*"As a single footstep will not make a path on the earth, so a single thought
will not make a pathway in the mind. To make a deep physical path,
we walk again and again. To make a deep mental path, we must think
over and over the kind of thoughts we wish to dominate our lives."*

Henry David Thoreau

Body Awareness Exercises to Achieve and Maintain Healthy Weight

BEFORE WE CAN HEAL OUR physical bodies, we must first heal our spiritual, emotional, and mental selves. When the blockages in spiritual, emotional and mental energies are removed, our energies flow freely. Freely flowing energy makes physical healing, whole body healing possible.

Most of my clients struggle with extra body weight and the health issues that accompany the weight. Excess body weight is a personal challenge that self-repairs when we first heal the soul and mind. Then the actual physical act of balancing body weight will be much easier. This Chapter is about just that: moving through the change and personal growth that promotes true healing on all levels.

If true weight was simply a balance between calories in and calories out it would be quite simple to achieve and maintain our true, healthy body weight.

Body awareness type exercise: Yoga, Breath Work, Tai Chi, Qi Gong, Tae Kwon Do, Meditation, Walking Meditation, etc., helps people gain control of their lives and feel at peace with everything and anything. Let me explain.

When we stop the constant chatter inside our heads and still our minds through mindfulness activities, body awareness exercises, we tend to make choices that are in alignment with what is best for our health. We can do this without feeling deprived. This is because we have now learned to live in the present moment and are aligned in body, mind, and spirit. Body awareness exercises bring this balance of body, mind, and soul to our whole being.

A cluttered, "chattery" mind and a body that is not aligned in mind, body, and spirit tend to make decisions based upon impulse and cravings. These choices are made without regard to what is best for long-term health.

I started practicing yoga in August 2000, thirteen years ago! When I think about it, I can see how it has changed my personal decision making process. I too struggled, for years, with those proverbial 15-20 extra pounds. I just felt a little too pudgy, uncomfortable in my clothes and my skin! At the time I was making decisions about food, sugar, goodies and food based on cravings and impulses. If I restrained myself, I felt the self-deprivation thing. If I indulged I felt guilty.

My yoga practice started thirteen years ago and led me to other body awareness exercises and the peaceful decision-making that evolves. I can now make choices that are out of self-satisfaction and self-healing. No longer is conscious thought needed for me to accomplish this on a deeper level; body, mind, and soul! Sure I still eat cake, the 100% whole food treats I make at home. I eat a small piece, I am happy, and I could not care a less about eating more now! No guilt, no deprivation, I just enjoy and move on with a smile.

Body awareness exercises teach us personal awareness and a new way of communicating with ourselves. Eating, exercising and healthy lifestyle choices are no longer about guilt and deprivation: "Oh, I was bad, I just can't do this, I don't have the will power." Body awareness exercises stop you from listening to that voice. It is not your true voice or your true self. You become aware of your true voice, your true self and live balanced and peacefully around food and healthy choices.

When we quiet our minds, we use our emotions to our advantage. When our minds are busy, our emotions use us.

Yoga is one of the four health and healing components of the Dr. Dean Ornish Program for Reversing Heart Disease. Dr. Ornish's program has been so successful it is now covered by many insurance companies! A quote from Dr. Ornish about his program: "When you start doing yoga, exercise, and eating well, most people feel so much better so quickly they want to stick with it. Yoga is more sustainable than taking a pill."

Clients give me a hard time when I suggest yoga, telling me that doing poses is not enough. "I can't lose weight doing yoga, I need to really push myself hard exercising everyday," is something I have heard many times. It is not the physical exercise of yoga that keeps one thin and fit. Although it certainly helps as the poses create strength, tone, flexibility, and balance in body, mind and soul. It *is* this integration that yoga 'yokes' together to create a fit body and balanced body weight from within. This is balancing the body from the inside out!

The benefits of strength, tone, balance, and flexibility are not just physical. Your mind and soul reap these same benefits. Herein lies how yoga helps balance your body weight; happiness in mind, body, and soul.

Another area to consider in mind, body, and soul healing, when your weight seems to be stuck in a rut, is how much and how often you exercise. Truly excess exercise can work against us in the weight loss game. The body sees excess exercise as stress. Stress is a known factor in the conservation of body weight. Our body sees the issue in this light: we might just need that extra body weight later. Our bodies, when stressed, hang onto those extra pounds with a death grip. Excess exercise is body stress.

I used to live under the 'more is more' exercise plan: lifting weights for an hour every day coupled with either 4-15 mile runs, 10-20 mile bike rides, 10-15 mile power walks, or hours of XC skiing. In the summer I would throw in long swims across rivers and lakes. When I exercised for hours I felt I had burned many, many calories and deserved to indulge a little. I had earned it, right?!

My over-exercise obsession has ended! I have embraced the 'less is more' plan and have since lost those proverbial pounds. I am sure a couple of those pounds were muscle from my days of weight lifting, but most was body fat. My point is that less *is* more. When we slow down and listen to our bodies, we eat better and exercise more consciously. Our lives become more balanced, more Whole Health focused and our bodies respond by balancing themselves.

Research into present day hunter-gatherer societies shows that these people who are busy all day with food gathering, do not burn more calories than modern day supermarket hunter-gatherers! Exercise is important because our bodies are meant to move. However, whole food choices, eating and moving to your personal needs is a better way to lose extra body fat and maintain a healthy lean to fat body ratio.

Change is defined as the process of becoming different, substituting one thing for another, biological metamorphosis, personal development especially if seen as personally "life-changing." **Consciousness** is awareness of one's own existence and behaviors, staying inwardly attentive and mindful. **Conscious change** involves will and deliberateness, altering self in an intentionally conceived manner.

When we discover that something we are doing in our lives no longer serves our higher purpose as a human, conscious change is how we evolve. When we discover that the lifestyle and food choices we have made, consciously or not, are not reflections of our higher selves, we move to make change.

We realize our bodies are not vibrating at our highest level of health, and we seek out ways to change this; to heal current symptoms and weight issues and to prevent lifelong degenerative diseases from interfering with our vibrant quality of life.

Remember that life is always for us! Life force energy is always moving towards the positive: health and healing. It is humans who tend to go against the grain of nature and turn this flow of energy against themselves. If you allow yourself to be in this flow, positive things will just happen.

Yoga, or any body awareness type exercise, aligns our bodies, our minds, and our spirits so we can then make life giving choices. Body awareness exercises help us to become normalized in our eating, to reach a pattern of whole food, whole health habits that are normal and healthy for us.

Normal, healthy eating habits that achieve and maintain a balanced and healthy body weight:

- Eat when hungry without shame, guilt or obsession. Food is a fuel and is used as such allowing the true pleasure of good food to be enjoyed.

- Choose foods that satisfy the needs at the moment and think consciously, not obsessively or with guilt, about what was eaten earlier and what may be eaten later to achieve a healthy balance.

- Eat with awareness of taste, smell, and fullness in the digestive tract. Slow eating and thoroughly chewing food is a great way to have awareness of satiation.

- You stop eating when you are full. When you are fully conscious of no longer feeling hungry, you stop eating. You do not wait until that "stuffed" feeling hits.

When you engage in a regular practice of body awareness exercises, these habits become a part of who you are. You live all aspects of your life, not just around food, for what is best for your higher good.

Change is an energetic force in our lives. All energy needs to flow freely so it does not get stuck or blocked. Blockages create illness. Let change flow like a divinely flowing river. Allow yourself to evolve with the energy of change in your life.

I was inspired by this excerpt from a Sammy Hagar song. I wrote it down, many years ago, because it spoke to me. I find it fitting here. I think the "darkness" he speaks of is a crisis we face that makes us change our lives. Whether the crisis is our personal crisis or a crisis we watch a loved one go through, it impacts us and moves us to make changes in our lives.

From the mouth of Sammy Hagar (see Mom, there is wisdom in rock and roll!): **"We've got to learn how to listen before we learn to talk, we've got to learn how to crawl before we learn to walk. And if you want a little peace, sometimes you've got to fight. We've got to walk through the darkness, before we stand in the light."**

I wish you well on your journey of self-exploration, healing, and ever-evolving change.

Chapter 8
Whole Health Lifestyle Choices

"It may be when we no longer know what to do, we have come to our real work, and that when we no longer know which way to go, we have begun our real journey."

Wendell Berry

I AM INCLUDING THESE HEALING, lifestyle choices as my bonus thoughts on healing. Each one could easily be a Chapter of its own. I choose to make them quicker suggestions for good reasons. Humans work best, making healthy changes to last their lifetimes, when we figure it out in the context of our own life experiences. We then have ownership of the wisdom.

I truly believe when each of us make the choice to eat better and exercise daily (outdoor exercise **is** best), we will intuitively want to add every healthy choice we can into our lives. Feeling good truly creates a ripple effect of wanting to feel better. The result is that we keep our personal health and healing energy flowing!

There are many more whole health lifestyle choices. I hope you use these suggestions to find your own path of healing lifestyle choices.

Chewing

"Drink your solids, chew your liquids."

Dr. John R. Christopher

The chewing process serves many functions. I always teach my students, young and old, about the importance of chewing. The chewing action sends messages between the mouth, brain, and stomach alerting your digestive tract that food is coming. This helps to jump start the whole digestive tract for smoother functioning by getting your digestive juices rolling!

Have you ever chewed a piece of gum only to find your stomach churning and growling within 20 minutes? Your chewing of gum is telling your tummy food should be coming. In the case of chewing gum, nothing is actually headed down to the stomach.

Chewing breaks food into smaller pieces for ease of swallowing and ease of digestion. Enzymes can digest these smaller pieces more efficiently.

Chewing mixes carbohydrate based foods with saliva. Saliva is rich in the enzymes that digest carbohydrates. Saliva makes the food you eat more alkaline, assisting with the gas issue discussed below.

Chewing is imperative for healthy digestion of carbohydrates. The more thoroughly chewed your carbohydrates, the less bloating and gas in your digestive tract. Bloating can be caused by carbohydrates that are not digesting well from inadequate chewing and inadequate mixing with saliva enzymes. You will literally stop digestion in its tracts from poor chewing habits making the stomach and small intestine work harder than nature intended.

Chewing is the beginning of carbohydrate digestion. Chewing breaks down complex carbohydrates and releases the natural sugars in the food. This releasing of the natural sugars in carbohydrates satisfies and tames your sweet tooth. You will have fewer sweet cravings as your body's need for sugars is better satisfied by the chewing and digestion of whole foods.

Chewing well releases all of the flavors in food. When your senses experience all the flavors in each meal, you will feel better satisfied. Flavor and sensory satisfaction prevent cravings.

Chewing breaks apart proteins and fats making the oils, proteins, vitamins, minerals, and ALL nutrients available for maximum absorption.

Chewing well and slowly prevents you from over-eating. Conscious chewing is a body awareness exercise that creates mindfulness! When you slowly chew your food, the messages relayed from mouth to brain, and brain to stomach are better heard and perceived by you. This means you will recognize the "full" feeling sooner and eat less.

Chewing food slowly and well promotes healthy balancing of body weight. Yes, you will lose weight when you are mindful about chewing!

Try this experiment: Eat a carrot. Chew it poorly, leaving good size chunks in your mouth and swallow them. Aim for the size of sunflower or pumpkin seed chunks and swallow. What do you think you will find in your solid waste? You've got it! Those very same chunks of carrot, unchanged.

Now eat another carrot, chewing it into the consistency of yogurt or pudding. Do you think you will find chunks of carrot in your solid waste? No! Your body will be able to digest and absorb all the nutrients it needs from that carrot because you chewed it into liquid mash.

"Drink your solids, chew your liquids." An intelligent saying Dr. John Christopher, Naturopath, repeated over and over in the classes I took in Natural Healing and Herbal Medicine. When the solid food you swallow is in liquid form from chewing, your body can absorb all the nutrients in that food. This ensures healthy cell regeneration and deposits into your nutritional bank, not nutritional withdrawal and the resultant degenerative cells! Remember healthy cell biology **is** the foundation of good nutrition and whole health!

When you consume liquids, chew them thoroughly. Do a fine job mixing those salivary enzymes with all that passes **slowly** through your mouth. Chewing liquids is an issue with the trend of eating liquid meals: smoothies. Most people blend up great food and then slug it down with no conscious thought of chewing. In order to digest properly, you need to chew those liquid foods. Chew your smoothies, take time and eat them slowly.

To slow down and enjoy meals try calming activities before you eat. Take the time to wash your hands and face with warm water. Sit down and take several slow, deep breaths. Focus on gratitude for those who brought this food to your table: farmers, farm hands, truck drivers, the cook (thank yourself if you are the cook!) and anyone else involved in the process of getting food to your table.

With each mouthful:

- chew at least 30 times
- put your eating utensils down after each bite
- experience the tastes, textures, colors, aromas, everything about your food
- enjoy conversation
- enjoy the peace if you are dining alone
- let chewing become a calming, meditative action

When you finish eating, resist the urge to bolt from the table to your next activity. Sit, linger, and give thanks.

Taking the time to chew will increase cellular health as the nutrients are more available to the cells! Enjoy every meal for the gift of life that it is.

Detoxing from Food "Drugs"

A food "drug" is anything we eat that we have no control over. Food is a "good girl drug."* I claim no gender bias; food can be the good guy drug too! Anyone who uses food to "medicate" themselves, medicate their emotional and spiritual needs, is using food as a drug. This means over-eating the food, craving it and all the negative thoughts and feelings that go along with this process. Eventually your body actually has a physical need for the food to feel "normal". This is not a healthy physical need but one that develops from continually altering the body cells' physiological functions with unhealthy foods.

Sugar, refined carbohydrates, and packaged, processed foods are our biggest addictive food drugs. The impact on the body's physiology is apparent in adult onset pre-diabetics and diabetics. Detoxing from food drugs takes commitment to a healthier lifestyle, which is what this book is all about!

Eat 100% whole food diet. This will immediately eliminate all the triggers: sugar, processed foods, refined foods, and anything artificial. Truly, this should be the end of the story: cold turkey switch to 100% whole foods. Your health problems will be solved and your body will heal.

But, there is always more to the story, so I will give you some more hints and tips.

* "good girl drug" is a concept handed to me from Kathy Montan
http://www.kathymontan.abmp.com/
Body-Centered Expressive Therapy, Canton, NY

Drink liquids that have no calories and no artificial sweeteners. This eliminates sodas, "vitamin drinks," sweetened ice tea, and fruit juices. Whole food eating excludes these drinks; obviously they are not whole foods.

Healthy liquids are water and herbal teas. Coffee and black or green teas do not have calories as long as you keep the sugar out. If you need a little sweetness in your coffee or tea, keep it natural. Find a good source of local, raw honey and use it sparingly.

Artificial sweeteners are not whole foods. Do not fool yourself into believing they are okay choices, your salvation from sugar addiction. They are marketed as such because they are making big money for companies. Artificial sweeteners are just that: artificial. They create health problems of their own. Learn to tame your sweet tooth and respect whole food sweeteners using them in serious moderation.

Avoid caffeine if you need to regulate your insulin and blood sugar, such as in the case of pre-diabetes and existing diabetes. Heal your body, then feel free to use caffeine, sparingly and with respect for the stimulant "drug" that it is.

Eat regular meals (whole foods) that are balanced in complex carbohydrates, protein, and fats. A plate of food could have a large pile of vegetables steamed or stir-fried, a small portion of whole grains if you tolerate them well, a small portion of lean meat from grass-fed animals or a serving of beans with some raw nuts and seeds mixed in. Add in a small piece of low sugar fruit for dessert.

Stop eating by 6 PM so your body is not trying to digest food while you sleep. Also, keeping your blood sugar and insulin levels down before bedtime helps with weight loss and healing. Now, I say this with caution as there are days when I do not eat three meals by 6 PM. If I am hungry I eat a whole food snack later than 6 PM and do not let it stress me. Then there are days I just do not eat three meals. So be it! Life is truly about balance.

I look to my dog's and four cats' wisdom. They eat and think nothing of taking a nap immediately after a meal. If their food is balanced, whole foods and they are not over-fed, they do not become overweight despite post-eating sleep.

Eat breakfast, making it healthy whole foods. Breakfast revs up your metabolism from the overnight "fast." Breakfast foods can be dinner left overs. Who said it had to be boxed cereal and milk? Cereals are highly processed food products. Pasture-raised, naturally fed chickens give healthy eggs. Have one of these eggs for breakfast with some fruit, maybe a slice of sprouted grain bread toasted with grass-fed butter and almond butter? I am merely throwing out thoughts and ideas. Think outside the box of the SAD: Standard American Diet. It is called "sad" for a reason; the Standard American Diet is killing us. Think whole food and healing! Eat whole foods and heal.

Or, skip breakfast and fast a little longer. My point is to know what works for your body. Some people do better without breakfast for many reasons. Maybe you are just not hungry in the AM. Perhaps eating in the AM starts the blood sugar surges that keep you wanting to eat all day. Whatever your body tells you, listen.

Get plenty of sleep. More on this later!

Exercise every day. Get outside and move your body, **fresh air and natural light are part of this process.** When you exercise, you feel better. People who feel better are more likely to make better food choices. Feeling good begets wanting to feel even better! It is a ripple effect! This is all about the alignment of body, mind, and spirit. See the previous Chapters on exercise and mind-body alignment!

Surround yourself with community, family, and friends, who support your path to health. Do not let others drag you down with their, "oh! Come on, just one bite won't kill you." Processed crap food <u>is</u> killing us as individuals and as a nation! Look around, a large segment of our population is overweight and under healthy, overfed and under nourished!

Be positive and upbeat. Be a healing role model for yourself and everyone! One who leads by actions, not preaching. Preaching health to uninterested family and friends is a losing battle. Trust me on this one. After twenty plus years, I gave up preaching and began teaching those who truly want to listen, learn, and change their lives. Let your actions and your resultant radiant health silently speak for themselves.

"We must find a way to replace yearning for what life has withheld from us with gratitude for what we have been given."

Ken Nerburn

Make **you** your priority!

You are not depriving yourself of anything but ill health. The side effects of whole food eating and whole health living are true health and healing, a body completely free of disease symptoms, feeling vibrant energy every day and geared for healthy longevity. Are there any prescription drugs with these side effects?

Healthy Gut Flora = Healthy Human

Promoting healthy gut flora is common knowledge among holistic healers. Gut health is now becoming more a part of mainstream thinking. The gut, and the gut's flora, is the seat of healthy immunity, healthy nervous system function, and healthy human bodies!

Healthy gut microorganisms help to create and maintain the body's various immune cells and keeps the immune system balanced. 80-85% of our immunity is located in the gut wall. It just makes good sense to maintain healthy gut flora!

Our gut flora help to: digest food so we can absorb and use nutrients; manufacture nutrients necessary for health and life; maintain healthy bowel function to avoid constipation or diarrhea; prevent digestive tract symptoms and illnesses; prevent invasion by pathogenic organisms; neutralize toxic substances; maintain a healthy nervous system (think about the saying "gut feeling"); and many, many more crucial functions in the human body. Healthy gut flora is essential to and synonymous with good health.

What compromises healthy gut flora? Some gut compromisers are:

Manufactured, processed "foods" are devoid of nutrition, they lack beneficial microbial flora and are high in sugar and refined grains that feed unhealthy gut bacteria. Unhealthy gut bacteria compete for space with and can destroy healthy gut bacteria. Manufactured "foods" are also high in chemicals that destroy healthy gut bacteria: preservatives, artificial flavors and colors, and food "enhancing" chemicals (MSG, etc.), to name but a few food additives.

Antibiotics destroy gut bacteria. Antibiotics are the prescriptions you take as well as in the food you eat such as factory farm-raised chicken, beef, pork, fish, and dairy. Antibiotics are also in hand soaps, hand-sanitizers, dish soaps, laundry detergents and household cleaners. Keep antibiotics out of your home and life unless you truly need them for a life-saving infection. Your gut and overall health will be better served.

Drinking chlorinated and fluoridated water

Aspartame and other artificial sweeteners destroy healthy gut bacteria

Genetically modified (GMO) foods disrupt normal healthy gut flora. The human body does not recognize GMOs as nature made foods because they are not!

Birth control pills, hormonal methods of birth control and some prescription drugs.

Chemicals used to grow produce in non-organic farming methods.

Stress: real and perceived stress.

Prescription and over-the-counter medications.

Environmental pollution, as we are the microcosm of the macrocosm. What pollutes the Earth pollutes your body and pollutes your gut.

How can I maintain or regain my healthy gut flora?

Eat WHOLE foods! Get rid of anything that nature did not make or animal products that were not raised naturally.

Do not use antibiotics unless it is a life-saving choice. Learn to use natural methods of healing. If you must use an antibiotic make certain to follow the course of antibiotic therapy with vigorous methods to re-establish healthy gut flora. See below.

Avoid factory-farmed meat and animal products as antibiotics are used in the animals feed. If the animals eat them, they are in the animal foods you eat.

Eat organic produce to avoid the chemicals used in non-organic farming.

Avoid genetically modified foods. They are NOT whole or natural, need I say more about how they disrupt gut flora?

Drink water that is pure, no chlorine or fluoride added.

Avoid antibacterial soaps, lotions, and hand-sanitizers. Learn natural ways to keep your immune system healthy.

Learn natural and non-hormonal methods of birth control. Synthetic hormones disrupt healthy micro-flora and have a host of other dangerous side effects.

Eat fermented foods: yogurt, kefir, real sour cream and cultured butter/buttermilk, sauerkraut, kimchi, and soft cheeses that were not heated.

Fermented foods that have been heated after fermentation no longer contain the gut enhancing bacteria. Canned sauerkraut is an example of a fermented food that is heated for preservation. The canning process is heat. The heat used to can the sauerkraut destroys the good microorganisms. Raw sauerkraut is not heated and thus maintains the healthy, gut-enhancing organisms.

Make healthy lifestyle choices around stress: exercise, time outside, getting natural sunlight and fresh air, avoiding the news as it is negative and stresses your very being, and avoiding negative people. FYI: Sun exposure is **not** bad, we need it to thrive. Over-doing sun and burning is not a healthy choice. Fifteen minutes of naked, full sun everyday would benefit body, heart, mind and soul!

Avoid medications unless absolutely necessary. There are natural ways to heal, making medications unnecessary.

Take probiotics. A brand I recommend, only because I have had personal success re-establishing healthy gut flora, is Pharmax. I advise using a whole food diet as your source of nutrients. However, after a round of antibiotics, a good probiotic supplement helps re-establish the normal gut flora to ensure gut health and overall whole body health. Then continue to maintain healthy gut flora with whole food eating.

Eat root vegetables grown in organic soil. Gently wash dirt off so you do not destroy all soil microbes and eat the peelings!

Avoid the known gut microbial killers, that I have mentioned, at all costs. Your gut health is your whole body health.

Raw apple cider vinegar contains the mother, the culture that ferments cider into vinegar. Use raw apple cider vinegar to make your own salad dressing, sprinkle over vegetables or use as a rejuvenating drink in water mixed with raw, local honey. See simple recipe in Chapter 10.

Fermenting your own vegetables is a great way to get healthy microbes into your Gastro-Intestinal tract. Here are some general guidelines:

1. Shred and cut your favorite vegetables into very small pieces.

2. Juice some celery to use as the brine. Celery is very high in natural sodium and keeps the fermenting vegetables anaerobic. This eliminates the need for adding sea salt. Salt prevents growth of pathogenic bacteria.

3. Pack the vegetables and celery juice along with the inoculants, the started culture. Pack the vegetables into a 32 ounce wide-mouthed canning jar. Pack them down well to eliminate all air pockets. Air turns fermentation from anaerobic to aerobic. Kraut pounder tools are available.

4. Top with a cabbage leaf, tucking it down the sides of the jar. Make sure the vegetables are completely covered with celery juice and that the juice is all the way to the top of the jar to eliminate trapped air.

5. Seal the jar and store in a warm, slightly moist place for 24 to 96 hours, depending on the food being cultured. Ideal temperature range is 68-75 degrees Fahrenheit; 85 degrees max, as heat will kill the microbes.

6. When finished fermenting, store vegetables in the refrigerator to slow down the fermentation process.

Caution: avoid eating the fermented vegetables out of the jar. You can introduce unwanted organisms into the jar. Use a clean spoon to take out what you're going to eat. Recap the jar with the vegetables covered in the brine.

Culturing your own foods is rather easy, especially once you get into the swing of things. Some people do not have the time or interest in home veggie fermentation. That is just fine! If you understand and appreciate the value of fermented foods, purchasing raw, fermented food works, too! Several companies make delicious versions for you! Try special ordering Deep Root Organics or Rejuvenate products from your local health food store or the health food section of your favorite supermarket.

Product names and information:

> Deep Root Organic Grated Beets
>
> Deep Root Organic Red Cabbage
>
> Deep Root Organic Grated Carrots
>
> Deep Root Organic Daikon Radish with ginger
>
> Deep Root Organic Green Cabbage Sauerkraut

I have tried them all, they are very yummy!

Another brand that can be special ordered is Rejuvenate. Information is:

> Rejuvenate Organic Kimchi
>
> Rejuvenate Organic Sauerkraut
>
> Rejuvenate Organic Vegi-Delite

Have fun eating good gut food!

Sleep

Sleep; eight hours of good sleep is a beautiful thing! People who are in bed and asleep before 10 PM sleep better and wake up more refreshed. This is because you are following the normal circadian rhythms of the body and the earth (remember we are a microcosm of the macrocosm). The body likes to be "normal!"

Avoid stimulating things like bright screens, computers, TV, cell phones and iPads, for two hours before bed. The bright light of "screens" simulates daylight and interferes with your melatonin production. Melatonin is the hormone your body produces so you sleep deeply and peacefully.

If you have trouble sleeping, examine your coffee and other caffeine containing food intake. Chocolate, teas, and sodas - yikes the sugar and artificial sweeteners in soda will also keep you awake! Cut back to 1-2 cups per day and consume in the AM or very early afternoon. You should see profound changes in your ability to get to sleep and sleep well all night.

Personally I would get rid of anything that is not real: soda, whether sugar sweetened or artificially sweetened. There is nothing whole food about soda.

I will give you a little inspiration to make certain you are getting enough sleep. Adequate sleep is important for many reasons. Adequate sleep slows aging! Learn what your body needs to feel refreshed, energetic and just plain good all day. Make certain you get this amount of sleep every night. Your health depends on it.

The body sleeps best when the sleep cycle starts before 10 PM and you get a solid seven to nine hours of sleep. Your bodily rhythms function best when they match the rhythms of the earth. This may sound too simplistic and tree-huggy; but truly we were meant to function with the cycles and flow of nature because, well, we are nature.

Our bodies have regular periods of higher energy, better digestive capability, and better sleeping efficiency. This is your body flowing with nature. Use this knowledge and help your body flow smoothly with nature, with itself.

Sleep's many benefits:

- Detoxes the body

- Repairs damage and inflammation, slowing aging!

- Decreases risk for cancer, autoimmune disease, cardiovascular disease..... many and any disease, as damage and inflammation are repaired during sleep, see above

- Your brain functions better, memory and intelligence are enhanced

- Lessens depression, anxiety, stress, any negative nervous system issue

- Keeps blood pressure, cholesterol, insulin and blood sugar levels in check

- Curbs cravings for unhealthy foods. When we are tired we reach for comfort foods which may not be the healthiest choices in a Whole Food, Whole Health lifestyle.

- Keeps your body chemistry, your hormones better balanced

- Adequate sleep promotes weight loss. Increase your sleep by 1 hour nightly, falling asleep before 10 PM, and you will shed ten to twenty pounds. Excess weight is a symptom of a body out of balance. The body functions best when its rhythm is natural!

Is this all sounding similar to the benefits of exercise? Truly, the benefits are the same because healthy choices create a healthy sequence of events in your glorious body! Cellular biology, Baby! We are back to that again!

Make it a personal goal to get plenty of good sleep, starting before 10 PM, every night!

Whole Food Supplements

Whole food supplements are supplements made from real foods, herbs, and nature's medicines. They are 100% whole, like the whole food diets nature intended us to eat!

Whole food supplements can be:

- whole herb herbal teas

- powdered whole herbs encapsulated

- whole herbal tinctures

- powdered whole foods like green food drinks; go to www. herbdoc.com and check out SuperFood Plus, this is an example of a whole food supplement

- whole food, fresh made juices; use in moderation as they are just the juice of the whole food; fresh juices are good for cleansing diets

- sea plants, also called sea vegetables or sea weeds

- whole herb and whole food oils, essential oils

- whole foods that are labeled as super foods: current examples are blueberries, raw cacao, etc. These are simply foods shown to be ultra high in nutrients, micro-nutrients, and phyto-nutrients.

Any whole food in their original, natural state are super foods. Foods as simple as heritage variety apples, beets, carrots, potatoes, squash, whole grains, etc. are all super foods! Science just has not picked them apart down to their phyto-nutrients and micro-nutrients to alert you, the consumer, that these heritage foods are super high in nutrients. Nature made them this way; of course they are super high in nutrients! Nature makes no mistakes!

If you choose your supplements the way you choose your food: whole substances like your whole food diet, you will be getting superior, natural nutrition. This is supplementation that has the full synergy of natural nutrients. Your body cells (genes) recognize them as real substances and know how to use these nutrients. We were designed to use whole foods, not refined parts of foods.

With all this said, when you have a nutritional deficiency, you may need to use nutritional supplements. If you had a magnesium or selenium deficiency, for example, supplementing can fix this deficiency. You want to get this single nutrient, for the correction of deficiencies, from a natural source, not a petro-chemical, lab created substitute. An example of good sources of minerals is whole herb products: teas and encapsulated whole herbs.

Why Your Body Prefers Whole Everything

Synthetic supplements are single chemical constituents. Nature meant for you to ingest foods in their whole form. This ensures you get the complete symphony of nutrients that are meant to work together. Everything works synergistically to make each individual part work better as a whole. We, as humans, do not have a clue what all those nutrients are in whole foods, whole supplements, and whole medicines. Knowing is interesting for satisfying curiosity but it does not change how they work in the body. When something you ingest is whole, all of the parts work together to create the nutritional and healing effect nature intended.

Your body only absorbs a small percentage of synthetic forms of vitamins and minerals - and it utilizes even less. Your body gets the best bio-availability when foods, supplements, and medicines are in whole food form!

When you put substances in your body that lack balance, these substances can then create an imbalance in your body. Supplements that are not whole create the same problems in the body as refined foods.

The nutrients in whole food, whole herbs and whole supplements work synergistically with each other to provide natural health benefits.

Read labels on supplements just as you would on foods. Strive to find supplements that are whole and lack synthetic additives. Avoid artificial flavors, colors, preservatives, and any ingredient that does not sound like it came from nature. When we strive to avoid food laden with unnatural substances, it only makes sense to hold our supplements to the same natural standards.

Potential Supplements to a Whole Food Diet

Whole food vitamin: Superfood Plus from **www.herbdoc.com** is my favorite choice. There are many whole food supplement powders on the market. Find one you like and use it. Again: read labels.

Vitamin D: Fifteen to twenty minutes of full body outdoor sun exposure daily takes care of your Vitamin D needs. Yes, that means naked sun time (if possible, of course)! Avoid sunscreens, as they prevent Vitamin D formation in your skin.

Natural Vitamin D is in pasture-raised egg yolks: skip the *egg whites only* mentality* and eat eggs as a whole food! Pasture-raised meat especially the liver, grass-fed cheeses, grass-fed butter, and cod liver oil are other natural Vitamin D sources.

Omega 3 and healthy fats: all the food items above have natural Omega 3 and healthy fat profiles.

Deep sea fish are a source of healthy fat. Avoid eating large predator fish as they are a storehouse for toxins. Predator fish are at the top of the food chain and have a heavier toxic load.

*Eggs (naturally raised) are good for you. Let your common sense prevail here, not corporate sponsored nutrition and health information. Eat the yolk and white, they work together synergistically to provide whole food nutrition.

Eat seaweed. Chlorella (chlorella is in the SuperFood Plus), hijiki, dulse, kelp.

Nuts and seeds: hemp seeds, walnuts, golden flax (omega 3 in flax are harder to utilize), any nuts and seeds. Eat and enjoy them raw and organic!

Magnesium is generally low in the foods we eat and needed for calcium to function in our bodies.

Natural sources of magnesium:

Legumes; including beans, peas, lentils, black beans and peanuts, and fermented soy such as tempeh, miso and natto are all respectable sources of magnesium.

Whole grain such as whole, *heritage* seed, wheat breads, pastas, and tortillas, brown rice, whole "hulless barley," whole rye, and other unrefined grains.

You should note that refined grains (white flour) are generally very low in magnesium and actually rob your body of minerals. When white flour is processed, the magnesium rich germ and bran are removed. Bread made from whole grain wheat flour provides more magnesium than bread made from white refined flour.

All green foods such as parsley, okra, collard greens, broccoli, kale, celery, plantain, spinach, romaine lettuce, dark leafy lettuces, dark greens and mustard greens are high in magnesium. Green vegetables such as spinach, and all those listed above, are good sources of magnesium because the center of the chlorophyll molecule (which gives green vegetables their color) contains magnesium.

*Heritage wheat is a more pure strain of wheat and has not been hybrid crossed many times. Heritage wheat strains are lower in gluten and far better tolerated by our bodies. If you have celiac disease, avoid all wheat. Heritage varieties are: Elkhorn, Spelt and Kamut.

Fish and seafood: All fish is a good source of magnesium. Good examples are: Halibut, Oysters, Rockfish, and Scallops.

Tap water can be a source of magnesium, but the amount varies according to your water supply. Water that naturally contains more minerals is described as "hard." "Hard" water usually contains more magnesium than "soft" water.

Northern NY water, where I live, tends to be high in calcium and lower in magnesium. Eat magnesium rich foods to fortify yourself!

Breath

Whole foods help your cells regenerate as healthy as or healthier than the original parent cell, not degenerate into a less healthy cell. Better breathing brings more oxygen to every cell, again helping to regenerate healthier cells. Your each and every breath is life giving. Learn to breathe deeply to increase the flow of oxygen into your body and exhale the waste carbon dioxide from your lungs.

Breathing Technique to improve your health!

This is a breathing technique recommended by Andrew Weil, an MD and a naturopathic trained physician who is a pioneer in the Integrative Medicine movement and an advocate of whole foods, whole health and natural living. What a guy!

Dr. Weil has used this technique with his patients for decades and claims practicing this breathing technique two times daily will create drastic changes in the body and improve your health. He calls it his low tech intervention! Dr. Weil says the original meaning of conspiracy is to breathe together; this is a conspiracy for better health! Breathe better and improve your health today and everyday!

Improvements he has seen in his patients include:

* stopping chronic digestive problems

- ending cardiac arrhythmias
- lowering blood pressure, decreasing inflammation in the body
- counteracts anxiety and panic disorders; increases feel good hormones in the body, balancing neurochemistry, promoting restful sleep
- increases circulation eliminating cold hands and feet, changes skin temperature

The first thing you want to determine is whether you are a chest or belly breather. My students in public school always loved this calming exercise. Lie down if you can, otherwise sit up straight. Place one hand on your chest, one on your belly. Breathe normally and determine which hand raises more, your hand on belly or your hand on chest. If you are a chest breather, consciously retrain yourself to breath with your belly. Belly breathing moves the diaphragm muscle, which sits below your lungs. When you breathe with your belly, the diaphragm muscles drops down farther and allows your lungs to fully expand. Nice big belly breaths everyone!

Simple calming breath:

Consciously make your breath *deeper, slower, quieter and more regular.* If you notice, when you are angry or stressed, your breathing is rapid, shallow, noisy and irregular. Slow down and calm your breath. You will calm your body, mind, and spirit.

Just consciously making your exhalation deeper will involuntarily make your inhalations deeper. This breathing habit automatically calms the body.

Use this simple, calming breathing technique: to take a break at your desk, when sitting in traffic, before reacting to a negative or stressful situation, when having a craving for something that is not whole food, or to relax and go to sleep.

Healing Breath Technique: To start, exhale very deeply.

1. inhale slowly and quietly, through the nose, to the count of 4

2. hold breath to a slow count of 7

3. exhale slowly and somewhat noisily through the mouth, counting to 8 as you exhale.

4. when exhaling, purse lips and press your tongue to the roof of your mouth, just behind the front teeth.

Repeat this for 4 inhale-exhale cycles 2 times a day. After a month increase to 6-8 inhale-exhale cycles 2 times a day. Never more than 8 cycles, 2 times a day.

Breathe deeply, today and every day, to gain better cellular health for life!

Common Scents-ability

Our consumer world is full of synthetic scents: laundry detergent and softeners, lotions, perfumes, soaps, deodorants, and all hair care items to name but a few scented products.

In most commercial products these scents are synthetic chemicals that are very concentrated and strong smelling. Most are petrochemicals.

Compare this to body care items scented with natural plant essential oils. Natural scents are subtler and less intrusive to our senses and the senses of those around us.

Here are some things to think about in regards to body care products and their scents:

When you are sporting several scented things on your body they tend to not blend well and their "smells" work together antagonistically. Think about your clothes and the scents from laundry care products mingling with the lotion you put on after you showered with a scented soap, the hair care products you use (including shampoo and conditioner), your scented deodorant and the perfume you then sprayed on. This is a lot of synthetic scents for the olfactory glands, liver, nervous system and all of your body cells to handle.

Synthetic scents are toxic to body cells. Repeated exposure has been linked to endocrine disruption and several types of cancer. On an immediate note, these scents are irritants to the nose, eyes, throat, skin, nervous system, truly your whole body. The scents are an irritant to your whole being and are irritants to all of the people with whom you come into contact with.

Synthetic fragrances have been linked to fetal abnormalities. Many people are chemically sensitive to these fragrances. Do you know people who cannot walk down the laundry product aisle because they literally get sick from the synthetic fragrances? Reactions can range from mild irritation to very severe allergic reactions.

Be aware of your scent impact on your health, the health of others and the planet as a whole. Opting for unscented, naturally scented, and products made with all-natural ingredients will help you, others you come into contact with, and the planet.

Remember, our bodies are but a microcosm of the macrocosm. What we do to ourselves we do to the earth. What we do to the earth we do to ourselves.

Carefully read the labels of the products you buy. If something is heavily scented, it is very wise to avoid it. Also avoid a product whose list of ingredients is a mile long and contains multiple unrecognizable chemical names. The product's front label may have the words "natural" and/or "organic" splashed all over it. When you investigate, by actually reading the ingredients list, you will find a whole different story unfolding. With most "natural'" products the ingredients are far from "natural" or "whole!"

Remember whole foods make us healthy. "Whole" products make everyone healthier. Use the same thought process with your body care products as you would with the food you put into your body; is this product "whole?" Would I eat all the ingredients in this product? If you would not eat it, you probably should think twice about putting it on your body. What goes on the skin goes into the body!

Be happy, be healthy, and smell good naturally!

Kindness Begets Happiness

"What wisdom can you find that is greater than kindness?"

Jean-Jacques Rousseau

"A merry heart doeth good like medicine; but a broken spirit drieth the bones."

Proverbs 17:22

Kindness to self and others creates good energetic vibrations. When you act kindly or are treated kindly your body cells respond in positive ways. Your immune system works more efficiently, your nervous system pumps out more feel good hormones, your digestive tract digests and flows smoothly. Your whole body functions better on a wave of kindness.

Maintaining a positive attitude, despite life's challenges and hardships is an act of kindness to self. A positive attitude creates a wave of feel good chemicals in your body. These chemicals will, in turn, make you feel good making a wave of positive thoughts. It is a positive catch 22!

Be the ripple effect of kindness in your world. Ride the wave and spread good health.

For more on kindness, return to the end of Chapter 2 and re-read the part on self-love.

Connect with Nature
(Remember, we are nature!)

*"The care of the Earth is our most ancient and most worthy,
and after all our most pleasing responsibility. To cherish what
remains of it and to foster its renewal is our only hope."*

Wendell Berry

*"Humankind has not woven the web of life. We are but one
thread within it. Whatever we do to the web, we do to ourselves.
All things are bound together. All things connect."*

Chief Seattle, 1854

When, as humans, we realize we are but equal to all life on Earth, our true healing begins. We are nature, just as all else on Earth is nature. Our realization of the equality of all of nature is a grounding reality. When we heal the Earth, we heal ourselves. So it goes, when we heal ourselves, we heal the Earth. We are but a microcosm of the macrocosm - Earth.

"Honor the sacred.

Honor the Earth, our Mother.

Honor the Elders.

Honor all with whom we

share the Earth:-

Four-leggeds, two-leggeds,

winged ones,

Swimmers, crawlers,

plant and rock people.

Walk in balance and beauty."

Native American Elder

Chapter 9
Jump Start Your Health

WHEREEVER YOU ARE IN YOUR life, however long you have been taking less than "Whole" care of your body, every step you take towards whole foods and whole health living will make lasting changes in your cellular and whole body health. Jump start your health now!

I often hear from people how overwhelmed they are in regards to making healthy changes in their lives. "I do not know where to start." "I can never be as "pure" as you." "It is so complicated I do not want to bother." "Doing the same thing I have always done is so much easier; the path of least resistance!"

My best advice is to go slow. Change does not have to happen *all at once, right now!* Take baby steps and incorporate a new healthy lifestyle choice each week or even every two weeks. If you do something consistently for two weeks, it will become a habit. Add a new change, a new habit every two weeks. Keep track of your goals and achievements. Six months later you can look back at where you started, how far you have come and where you are right now and be utterly amazed at how small changes can add up to big changes in your health and life.

Start today by adding one more fresh fruit or vegetable to your daily diet. Enjoy the juicy, fresh taste!

Whole Health Lifestyle
Easy Steps to a Whole Health You!

Whole Foods are essential to nourish, prevent, heal and restore health. Drastically reduce, better yet eliminate, processed, packaged, or factory-made food. This includes fast food restaurants and frankly, most food at area restaurants. If not made from "fresh, whole" ingredients... back away from the table and politely excuse yourself! This simple act will rid your body of refined white flour, refined white sugar, artificial sweeteners, cheap vegetable oils, corn syrup, corn sugar, and synthetic ingredients of all types. **Start by increasing your intake of fresh, local and seasonal fruits and vegetables. Increase your intake of local greens: salad greens in the spring, summer and early fall, dark, heavy greens in the late fall and winter. Kale, collards and Swiss chard are examples of dark, heavier greens.**

Whole Supplements: Supplements you take to enhance your nutrition should also be whole substances. Whole food supplements help to address nutritional deficiencies. Highly processed and synthetic vitamins or minerals are not whole health substances. Seek out a qualified herbalist or naturopath who uses whole food supplements.

Water: Increase your intake of water: clean, pure water! If your water supply is chlorinated, filter it. Use a chlorine shower filter so you are not absorbing and breathing in chlorine as you shower. Filtering will also help you avoid the added fluorine or fluoride.

Daily physical activity: Start now, and continue some activity for life. Get outside and move. Fresh air and natural light are imperative to good health, endorphin, hormone and neurotransmitter production.

Maintain your social and intellectual integrity: Surround yourself with people who are positive thinkers and will enhance your positivity! Social connections keep us alive from the inside out. Keep learning new things throughout life to keep your neural pathways stimulated and healthy. Learn a new language, to play an instrument, take up an art form. Read and learn for lifetime mental, intellectual and neural health.

Get plenty of sleep! Skimping on sleep to "get things done" is not a whole health habit! Getting to sleep before 10 PM maximizes production of melatonin and works with the earth's circadian rhythms for great sleep and health. Stay away from bright lights and screens (computers, etc.) for at least two hours before sleep. Bright lights make your body think it is daytime and impair the sleep cycles. Get all lights out of the sleep area; even LED lights disturb good sleep hormone production. The moon and stars are fine!

Daily exposure to natural sun light and fresh air. Exercise, work, play, read, and relax outside!

Stress: A part of life, stress makes things happen. Interpret stress as a eustress, not distress. Eustress - this is good stress, positive stress, that which motivates! Learn stress neutralizing techniques and use them daily: yoga, meditation, breath techniques, exercise and time outside, art, music and dancing, singing, hot baths, massages. Embrace life; it is the only one you have right now!

Decrease use of chemical medicines: Decrease use of both prescription and over the counter drugs. The side effects are toxic and hard on the body. Living a whole health, whole food lifestyle will create radiant health naturally. A healthy body does not need factory made, laboratory created, chemical medicines. The body *knows* nature, *is* nature and responds best to natural substances.

Increase your use of organically grown and raised foods. This simple act helps to remove more chemical toxins from your life (and the Earth!). If you buy from local farmers, you can ask them directly how they raise their produce and animals. This is the best you can get for your body and health! **Buy the best quality food that your budget allows.**

Use chemical free body care: Chemical free products on skin, hair, and arm pits. If you would not eat it, you should avoid it topically.

All your thoughts and actions feed your body, heart, mind, and soul. Keep them whole and pure like your food. Decrease your exposure to negative media: TV, radio, newspapers, and internet news is all negative food.

You are only one workout away from a good mood!

Live **whole**, eat **whole**, and love yourself and others **whole**!

Be happy!

Paula's End Note:

Health and healing is not about perfection. It is about listening to yourself, your inner wisdom, and giving yourself what you need to balance body, mind, and soul.

May you find your true inner wisdom, your true balance.

To sum it all up, a statement well said by my dear friend, Rob Sachno:

"Life is interesting, entertaining. Don't take it seriously, that's the secret."

Perhaps that **is** the secret!

Much Whole Food and Whole Health LOVE!! Paula

Chapter 10

Whole Food Recipes to Live By and Love!

I OFFER THESE RECIPES, IN no particular order, as inspirations to get you into your Whole Food Kitchen playing with local, seasonal food. Any recipe can be a Whole Food recipe, any cookbook a Whole Food Cookbook. Using the principles outlined in Chapter 2 and 5, simply convert the recipe. One of my favorite cookbooks is an old Betty Crocker Cookbook that was my Grandmother's. I convert every recipe into a 100% whole food recipe. So hang on to all cookbooks you like and learn to convert!

Tourlou: Greek Veggie Mixed-Up

This makes a lot of vegetables. Change the amounts to suit your needs, or use the leftovers for breakfast and lunch. Yummy with scrambled eggs or spread on buttered whole grain toast.

Preheat oven to 350° F

> 5-6 zucchini
>
> 3-4 medium potatoes, heritage preferably, not hybrid white potatoes
>
> 2 large eggplants
>
> I quart canned tomatoes or lots of fresh tomatoes

3-4 cloves garlic, you will crush into the vegetables before cooking

1 large onion cut into big chunks

2-3 bay leaves

½ cup cold pressed olive oil

dash of nutmeg and thyme

1-2 cloves fresh garlic, press and stir into hot vegetables just before serving

Cut up everything and throw into a large, or two large, baking pans. Mix everything very well. Pour ½ – 1 cup water over each pan. Bake for 1 hour. Set timer for every 20 minutes. Open oven and mix vegetables adding more water as needed to keep vegetables from drying out. Mixture will be creamy and heavenly when finished.

Serve with chick peas, chicken, fish, beef or lamb dishes and 100% whole grain pita bread (even better is Food For Life Sprouted grain tortillas cut into quarters and toasted to crispy perfection. Use the ¼ pieces to scoop up the tourlou and chickpeas.

I have used many other vegetables with this, always in the base of tomatoes and eggplants: green beans, yellow squash, delicata squash, winter squash (butter cup and butter nut.) Truthfully, I do not even peel the winter squash. The skin softens nicely when cooking!

Spring Asparagus Recipe

bunch of asparagus, enough for whoever you are feeding

fresh oregano, if you have access to any

pasta tomato sauce seasoned with herbs: rosemary, thyme, oregano, parsley, basil.

local, grass-fed ground beef or Italian sausage for the sauce, optional

cooked chick peas

Parmesan cheese to grate

Lightly steam the asparagus spears, by this I mean they should remain bright green and very crisp. I put the large spears in first and steam for 1 minute (yes, I time it!), add the medium spears for 1 minute more and then the tiny spears for 1 last minute. The biggest spears get 3 minutes, tops.

Drain spears, save water in a mug and drink!

Put spears on plate and slice the length. Big ones I slice in ½ length wise and then slice them again so I have quartered the spears length wise. Medium spears also get quartered, tiny spears just ½.

Lay the spears on individual serving plates and slather with pasta sauce to please your palette.

Sprinkle approximately ½ cup cooked chick peas (or other white bean) over the spears and sauce.

Sprinkle grated Parmesan cheese to your taste.

Break up the fresh oregano, just pinching apart the leafs into 2 pieces and sprinkle over the top.

Enjoy. This is also good with no meat pasta sauce and beans, no meat pasta sauce and chicken pieces, no meat pasta sauce and fish as a side dish..... use your imagination in the kitchen!

If you are not an asparagus fan, do the same with fresh spring green beans or fresh spring peas you eat with the shell intact. Remember to only steam them lightly and drink the steam water, there are minerals in that water! Good for your bones, your body cells.

Paula M. Youmell, RN, MS, CHC

Bean and Nut Butter Burgers

1 medium onion, minced, or green onions in spring and summer

2 cloves garlic, minced or pressed

3 cups cooked beans of choice (kidney, black, chick pea, pinto. Learn to soak and cook your own beans, they are far better textured and tasting!)

½ cup natural peanut butter, organic (Arrowhead Mills is my #1 choice)

1/3 cup organic ketchup or tomato paste (organic avoids the corn syrup and crap ingredients, paste avoids all added sugars)

½ to 1 cup whole grain flour: oat, corn, buck wheat, amaranth, millet, quinoa.

Some of this flour can be oat flakes to make the burgers "heartier." You will have to play with amounts to get the right consistency so the bean mix is easy to work with to form into burgers.

Spices: I use 1 ½ tsp. each of cumin, coriander, turmeric and chili powder. I throw in curry powder if I have it, sort of redundant but I like spice.

Other options are Italian spices: rosemary, thyme, oregano, parsley, basil, marjoram...

Create your own spice blend, have fun with the process, eating included! I bet a cinnamon, cardamom, ginger, vanilla, and nutmeg blend would be snappy and fun!

Sauté onion and garlic in olive oil or pasture-raised butter. Mash or food process the beans. Add all other ingredients and mix well. Form into patties and fry as you would meat burgers. Dress as you like and serve!

The mix also works well as a raw bean spread on toast or for vegetable dipping.

You can also form this mix into smaller, falafel sized patties and bake or broil in the oven.

Paula M. Youmell, RN, MS, CHC

Curried Chick Peas

 2 cups dry chickpeas

 1 to 1 ½ cups organic tahini (sesame seed butter)

 2-4 cloves garlic, minced or pressed

 2 tbsp. low salt organic soy sauce or Bragg's Amino Acids

 ¼ cup chopped fresh cilantro

 ¼ cup chopped fresh basil

 ½ tbsp. fresh chopped thyme

 ¼ tsp. cardamom

 ¼ tsp. nutmeg

 2 tbsp. toasted sesame oil

Save the bean water after cooking. You can drizzle small amounts into the dish to make it less pasty and easier to mix everything

Optional ingredients: ½ to 1 cup finely chopped peanuts, ½ cup finely chopped dried cherries (raisins work well, as cherries are not always easy to find), ¼ cup un-hulled sesame seeds.

Cover beans with water and soak overnight in pot so they are in darkness. Change the soak water in the morning and cover and soak for another 24 hours. Soaking in darkness prevents bitterness and the soaking for 48 hours makes them easy to cook in 1 hour 15 minutes-- not 4 hours! You can drain and cover and soak for another 24 – 48 hours, and then use the beans raw as sprouted beans, making this into a raw, sprouted bean dish. In that case, do not cook the beans at all.

Put cooked (or raw, sprouted) beans in large bowl. Add the tahini, soy sauce, sesame oil, garlic and spices. Mix well, adding the bean soak - cook water to loosen things up as needed.

Add the peanuts, sesame seeds and cherries to add some interesting flavors.

Serve over a cooked whole grain rice or 100% whole grain pasta with a seasonal raw salad and voilà... dinner!

Sprouted Chickpea Hummus

First, I must confess, I am not good with exact measurements. I truly throw good food together in a pinch of this, handful of that method. I get ideas by reading cookbooks like novels and then start tossing things together that sound compatible. So this is a rough recipe, play with it!

approx. 1 to 1 ½ cups dry chickpeas and water to soak

approx. ½ - ¾ cup raw, un-hulled sesame seeds

approx. ¼ cup lemon juice

2-3 tbsp. raw, cold pressed sesame oil or olive oil

1-4 garlic cloves, finely chopped

½ cup fresh parsley, finely chop before putting in food processor

Optional: Add to your taste or liking unrefined sea salt, pepper, green onions or chives.

Optional spices: To give it a bit of a Mid-Eastern curry flair, try cumin, coriander and turmeric. Add after blending to your taste.

Food processor or Vitamix blender www.vitamix.com

Dry bean prep:

1. Put dry beans in a stainless steel pot with solid cover (glass covers allow light in and will make for bitter beans)

2. Cover with water and pot cover, set aside for 24 hours

3. Drain, rinse and recover with water in AM for 3-4 days to get a good soaking and sprouting

Assembling raw hummus:

1. Drain and grind beans in food processor

2. Grind sesame seeds in small amounts in a coffee grinder or blender. Do not grind in the food processor.

3. Add ground sesame seeds to food processor

4. Add rest of ingredients to food processor and grind like crazy! Be mindful of a potential hot, burning motor smell!

5. Add a tablespoon of water to make grinding easier and the hummus creamy to your liking

Sprouted, raw hummus will be a grainier texture than cooked chickpea hummus, unless you have a Vitamix blender. If so, add a bit more water to the Vitamix and the mix will grind more smoothly.

Serve with: cut up raw vegetables, 100% whole grain pita, Food For Life Sprouted Grain Tortillas

Broccoli and Cauliflower Salad

I take a head of broccoli and cauliflower each, rinse them well and cut them up into bite size pieces. I even use the stems (the nutrients are drawn up from the ground through the stem; they must be loaded with good stuff!)

Put all pieces in a glass dish that has a tight fitting cover. Make the olive oil and apple cider vinegar dressing that is listed under the salad dressing recipes. Coat the pieces well and refrigerate. I take it out and stir it up several times over the course of the day so it melds the flavors well. Marinating the vegetables this way does something to them that is different than cooking.

I also add seasonal vegetables to this: spring peas with or without the shells, asparagus, sweet and/or hot red peppers, etc.

I do the same thing with asparagus and roasted red peppers. I sometimes slightly steam the vegetables too, truly just slightly so they are still very bright in color and very crunchy.

Another dressing I use is basically the same except uses plain, unsweetened yogurt instead of the olive oil and vinegar. Depending on the yogurt, you may have to thin it out a little bit with water or milk. Also, play with the spices. You may find you need more spice in the creamy yogurt version than the oil and vinegar version.

I have added things like: raisins, nuts, seeds, etc. Pick extra ingredients that sound good to you.

Paula M. Youmell, RN, MS, CHC

Quick and Easy Bean Dinner Entree

Food For Life Sprouted Grain Tortillas. Tear them into quarters and toast on medium. They get crispy and delightfully delicious!

Put a pile of cooked beans (pinto, kidney, black, chickpea, etc.) and grated cheese on your plate.

Scoop with tortilla quarters and enjoy an easy meal.

Variation: spread beans and sprinkle cheese on the whole tortilla and put under the broiler for 2-3 minutes to melt cheese.

Enjoy with a plateful of local vegetables, raw or lightly sautéed.

Bulghur Wheat Tabouleh

1 cup bulghur wheat

2 cups boiling water

½ cup scallions, chopped

5 tbsp. fresh mint, chopped

2 medium tomatoes, seeded and chopped

2 medium cucumbers, chopped

1 cup fresh parsley, chopped (I add a lot of parsley, the more the better!)

5 tbsp. cold pressed extra virgin olive oil

6 tbsp. fresh lemon juice (I often use bottled, organic)

½ tsp. unrefined sea salt

½ tsp. fresh ground black pepper

Pour the bulghur in a bowl and add bowling water. Stir and cover bowl, let sit for 35 minutes. Drain the bulghur and squeeze out excess water. Use strainer or squeeze in your hands. Drink the water; always be thinking about the nutrients!

Add the remaining ingredients and toss gently.

Add chick peas, feta cheese, and black olives to make a yummy summer salad.

Serve with a side of chicken, fish...lamb!

Lamb Roast

oven at 325° F

Serve with garlic mashed potatoes and green salad or root veggie and cabbage slaw in fall or winter.

Place lamb in roasting pan. Slit the top in many places and add slices of fresh garlic or sprinkle with garlic powder (not garlic salt). Sprinkle liberally with rosemary, thyme and especially oregano.

Internal Temperatures:

To determine if lamb is done, take the internal temperature with a meat thermometer at the center of the roast. Degree of Cooking, Internal Temperature: Rare 140° F, Medium 150° F, Well done 160° F

Lamb Curry This is also very simple.

Using ground lamb or stew type chunks, stir fry the meat with curry spices and remove from pan.

Stir fry chunks of potatoes with skins on, carrots and onions. When vegetables are tender but still have a crunch, stir in meat and serve with green salad, cole slaw, or root veggie slaw, depending on the season and local availability.

Chicken Lo Mein

1 lb. chicken cut into thin strips

4 tsp. rapadura or sucanat sugar, divided

4 tbsp. apple cider vinegar

1/2 cup soy sauce or amino acids, divided

1 1/4 cups chicken broth

1 1/4 cup water

2 tbsp. toasted sesame oil

1/2 tsp. ground black pepper

3 tbsp. cornstarch

1 (16 ounce) package uncooked linguine, **whole grain** pasta

2 tbsp. sesame oil, divided

3 tbsp. minced fresh ginger root

2 tbsp. minced garlic

1/2 pound fresh shiitake mushrooms, stemmed and sliced

6 green onions, sliced diagonally into 1/2 inch pieces

3 peppers: yellow, red, orange

In a medium, stainless or glass bowl, combine the chicken with 2 1/2 teaspoons of unrefined sugar, 1 1/2 tablespoons vinegar and 1/4 cup soy sauce. Mix this together and coat the chicken well. Cover and let marinate in the refrigerator for at least 1 hour.

In another medium bowl, combine the chicken broth, water, sesame oil and ground black pepper with the remaining sugar, vinegar and soy sauce. In a separate small bowl, dissolve the cornstarch with some of this mixture and slowly add to the bulk of the mixture, stirring well. Set aside.

Cook the linguine according to package directions, drain and set aside. Heat 1 tablespoon of the vegetable oil in a wok or large saucepan over high heat until it starts to smoke. Add the chicken and stir-fry for 4 to 5 minutes, or until browned. Transfer this and all juices to a warm plate.

Heat the remaining vegetable oil in the wok or pan over high heat. Add the ginger, garlic, mushrooms, peppers and green onions, and stir-fry for 30 seconds. Add the reserved sauce mixture and then the chicken. Simmer until the sauce begins to thicken, about 2 minutes. Add the reserved noodles and toss gently, coating everything well with the sauce.

Serve and enjoy! Serves 2-4 depending on appetite and what else is being served to compliment this dish.

Simple Kale or Collards

   I bunch kale or collard greens

   I medium to large purple onion

   sweet potatoes (enough to feed the family)

   sesame oil or butter

cut potato into thin slices or small chunks

chop onion

cut greens into thin strips and the stems into tiny chunks

Melt butter and quickly stir fry green strips until just wilted, remove to bowl and cover.

Add onion, stem pieces and potato chunks and stir, cover and simmer for 5 minutes stirring every 2 minutes or so. When potatoes are tender but not mushy, add to bowl with greens.

Sprinkle with amino acids and serve.

You can also add curry powder or Chinese 5 spice to taste.

Optional Sweet curry sauce: dried prunes chopped, water, curry

Blend in the blender into a thin, sweet curry liquid and pour over vegetables. Mix and serve.

Fruit and Veggie Dips and Dressings
Apple Yogurt Dip

This is a great way to enjoy apple slices all fall and winter. OK, maybe not those fresh, local apples in August and September! Just enjoy their fresh taste.

> 1/3 - ½ cup plain, unsweetened yogurt
>
> 1-2 tbsp. nut butter (peanut butter, almond, hazelnut…)
>
> ¼ tsp. vanilla extract
>
> ¼ tsp. cinnamon (pinches of nutmeg, ginger, cardamom are also good)
>
> ¼ to ½ tsp. raw, local honey or maple syrup if you need it. Vanilla and cinnamon may be enough flavor.

Mix well. Add raw nuts or seeds to add some crunch, if you like. Sunflower seeds, pumpkin seeds, almond slivers, pine nuts, pistachios…

Cut an apple in 8 to 10 slices, dip and enjoy.

Veggie Dressings

When summer is on your door step, these healthy dressings will complement the abundance of healthy, fresh, local vegetables making eating a taste tempting experience. Enjoy these dressing recipes!

Creamy Yogurt Salad Dressings

You can re-create any flavor of creamy salad dressing using plain, unsweetened yogurt. Making homemade dressings is a great way to avoid commercial products. Read the labels, they are scary. Most commercial dressings are made with cheap vegetable oils and GMO ingredients.

Do not make huge quantities at a time unless you will use them up within a week or so. Foods without preservatives will get moldy far quicker than commercial products. These dressings all taste best when given one hour for the flavors to meld. Enjoy them on salads or as dips for veggie sticks and chunks!

Russian Dressing

1 cup yogurt

1 tbsp. tomato paste and apple cider vinegar

2 tbsp. Tabasco sauce

1 tbsp. each finely chopped celery and onion

1 tsp. Worcestershire sauce (read ingredients and purchase a natural one)

¼ tsp. unrefined sea salt

Blend all ingredients together well.

Thousand Island Dressing

1 cup yogurt

¼ cup Tabasco sauce

2 tbsp. pimento stuffed olives, minced

1 hard-boiled egg, chopped

2 tbsp. each scallions, green pepper, parsley finely minced

¼ tsp. each paprika and black pepper

Blend all ingredients well.

Roquefort Dressing

This is a French sheep's milk blue cheese, if you prefer, substitute your favorite blue cheese.

1 cup yogurt

2 tsp. raw apple cider vinegar

¼ tsp. cayenne pepper and sea salt

fresh ground black pepper to taste,

½ cup Roquefort cheese, crumbled

Blend all ingredients well, except the cheese. Gently fold in cheese.

Creamy Dressing for Pasta Salads (or green salads)

3 tbsp. apple cider vinegar

6 tbsp. organic cold pressed extra virgin olive oil

½ tsp. sea salt

½ tsp. fresh ground black pepper

1 scallion, chopped

2 tsp. Dijon style mustard (yellow also works well)

2 cloves garlic, minced

1 cup plain yogurt

basil and oregano to taste, 1 tsp. each or so…

Mix everything together except the yogurt, blend well. Add yogurt.

Caesar Dressing

2 small garlic cloves, minced

1 tsp. anchovy paste (optional and found near the tuna fish in the supermarket)

2 tbsp. freshly squeezed lemon juice, from one lemon

1 tsp. Dijon mustard and 1 tsp. Worcestershire sauce

1 cup plain yogurt

1/2 cup freshly grated Parmigiano-Reggiano

1/4 tsp. salt

1/4 tsp. freshly ground black pepper

In a medium bowl, whisk together the garlic, anchovy paste, lemon juice, Dijon mustard and Worcestershire sauce. Add the yogurt, Parmigiano-Reggiano, salt and pepper and whisk until well combined. Taste and adjust to your liking.

Ranch Dressing

I cup plain yogurt

½ tsp. each: chives, parsley, dill

¼ tsp. each: garlic and onion powder

1/8 tsp. sea salt and black pepper

Mix ingredients well and enjoy!

French Dressing

I cup plain yogurt

½ cup organic ketchup (no corn syrup)

¼ cup finely chopped onion (green onions in the spring is a fun variation)

I tsp. sea salt

I ½ tsp. Worcestershire sauce (read labels and buy all natural)

¼ tsp. garlic powder (more to taste if you like garlic)

1-2 tbsp. apple cider vinegar, add slowly to the consistency you want

Mix ingredients together. Slowly add the vinegar last.

To Dress or Not to Dress, Naked or Not is the Question!

Use all these dressings on leafy green salads, raw vegetable sticks and pieces, lightly sautéed or steamed vegetables. I am not necessarily advocating always slathering your vegetables. Learn to enjoy the fresh, wonderful taste of naked vegetables. With that said, dressing them up can be a fun change of taste, too!

French Onion Dip for Vegetable Sticks

If you read the ingredients in dry soup mixes, it is easy to replicate and avoid the fillers and synthetics.

Commercial Onion Soup and Dip Ingredients:

Onions (dehydrated salt, cornstarch, onion powder, sugar, corn syrup, hydrolyzed soy protein, caramel color, partially hydrogenated soybean oil, mono-sodium glutamate, yeast extract, natural flavors, disodium inosinate, disodium guanylate.

To make your own:

> 1 cup plain yogurt
>
> dry onions (spice section)
>
> onion powder
>
> garlic powder
>
> 1-2 tbsp. olive oil, if desired
>
> salt and pepper to taste

finely chopped fresh parsley, cilantro, or other fresh herbs you like

Enjoy dipping your vegetables without the added synthetics in manufactured products!

Homemade Olive Oil Mayonnaise

> 1 tsp. dry mustard
>
> 1 tsp. salt
>
> 2 -3 egg yolks, local eggs from free-range chickens are best
>
> 1 tbsp. boiling water

I cup olive oil, preferably organic, virgin and cold pressed

I tbsp. lemon juice

I tbsp. raw, local, apple cider vinegar

Blend salt and dry mustard in bowl. Whip egg yolks and blend in the above dry ingredients. Whip while gradually adding the boiling H2O. Add olive oil I TBSP at a time beating gently and constantly until ½ cup is used.

Now slowly drizzle the other ½ cup of olive oil while continuing to blend. Add lemon juice gradually and mix well. Add vinegar last while still mixing

I make this in a blender on low speed. You can also hand whisk it. Follow the steps exactly or it will not coagulate into mayonnaise. Trust me. I tried! I thought I would save time and just dump it all in the blender together. I did not get mayonnaise.

Use as you would commercial mayonnaise feeling good that you are missing out on the cheap, unhealthy GMO soy and canola oils and all the other unhealthy ingredients.

Refrigerate and use in two weeks or so. Works well for salads, sandwiches, and even chocolate mayonnaise cake. This is a very moist and yummy whole food cake. (Recipe follows in a few pages.)

I have used the following unrefined oils to make mayonnaise: raw sesame oil (not the toasted sesame oil as the flavor is very strong), sunflower oil, rice bran oil, and walnut oil.

Bran Muffins

2 cups whole grain flour, I use 2 to 3 different whole grain flours

1 tbsp. baking powder

½ tsp. salt

¾ cup bran flakes (get a whole grain, unsweetened brand)

2 tbsp. dark maple syrup (or use 1 large, very ripe banana, mashed well)

2 eggs from naturally raised chickens

1 cup milk

¼ cup plus 2 tbsp. melted butter, pasture-raised/grass-fed

2 tsp. cinnamon

¾ tsp. nutmeg

3 tsp. real vanilla

Oven at 350° F

Stir dry ingredients together. Beat maple syrup, egg, milk, and butter. Add wet and dry ingredients. Mix just enough to wet all the dry ingredients.

Fill muffin tins ¾ full and bake for 20 minutes.

Using a banana instead of maple syrup will obviously change the flavor to a banana – bran muffin. Yummy!

Ice Cream Substitute

I often am asked about ice cream as many people cannot resist the creamy, sweet, cool taste sensation of this treat. "What can I do to replace ice cream?" I have clients who eat it every night and know they need to end their ice cream relationship!

This is my version of something that is a creamy and yummy treat.

> ½ to 1 cup of whole fat, pasture-raised yogurt
>
> 1-2 tbsp. of organic peanut butter, almond butter, etc. (use some yummy nut butter to add to the creamy texture)
>
> ½ to 1 tsp. real vanilla extract.
>
> ½ to 1 tsp. raw, local honey or local maple syrup (the darker B and C grades of syrup are less refined and more nutritious)

Optional spices and flavors: cinnamon, cardamom, nutmeg, ginger, hazelnut extract, almond extract, coffee extract, chocolate extract or cocoa powder. Use your imagination and flavor to your liking.

Optional additions: raw, organic nuts and seeds of various types to give it crunchiness; organic no added sweetener granola; local and seasonal berries or fruit (depending on the time of year).

If I am eating this as breakfast, I often will beat a local, free-range, naturally-fed chicken egg and add to the yogurt-nut butter base then add flavors and fruit. The egg adds healthy fats, protein, vitamin A and D, iron, minerals and all sorts of good nutrients!

Caution: I would never use commercial eggs from the grocery store, factory farm-raised or organic varieties. I know the eggs I have available to me are from healthy, naturally-raised chickens. I know how the farmers care for their chickens and farm. Get to know your farmers; you just may make some of the best friends of your life!

French Breakfast Pastry Puff

These are yummy, little muffins my mom used to bake. *They taste like donuts without the deep frying!* Although I must confess, I am not above making 100% whole grain, whole food donuts and I fry them in home rendered lard from naturally fed and raised pigs. My kids enjoy them and I do, too! Email me for the recipe: pyoumell@gmail.com

> 1/3 cup butter (I use more like ½ cup)
>
> 1/3 cup sugar (I reduce to ¼ cup)
>
> 1 large egg, beaten
>
> ½ cup milk
>
> 1 ¼ cup flour (oat, corn, teff, quinoa, millet, amaranth, any 100% whole grain flour)
>
> 1 ½ tsp. baking powder
>
> 1 tsp. nutmeg
>
> ½ tsp. cinnamon
>
> Optional topping ingredients: sugar, cinnamon, melted butter

Preheat oven to 350° F.

For bigger muffins, use a six hole muffin pan, for smaller 'puffs' use a 12 hole muffin pan. Use melted butter to grease the muffin tins.

Melt butter and stir in sugar, beaten egg, and milk. Add dry ingredients and mix well.

Pour into 6 or 12 muffins. Bake 6 for 30 minutes, bake 12 for 20 minutes. They should be brown, pass the knife insertion test, and have a fabulous aroma to let you know they are finished baking!

Dip the tops in melted butter and roll in cinnamon sugar as an option. They are also delicious left plain!

Chocolate Mayonnaise Cake

Preheat oven to 350 F

Grease 8x8 or 9x9 pan, I use the home-made mayo to grease

> 2 cups whole grain flour
>
> 1 cup unrefined sugar, I reduce to ½ cup
>
> 1 tsp. baking soda
>
> 1 tsp. baking powder
>
> 6 tbsp. cocoa powder
>
> 2 tbsp. fat (use extra mayo)
>
> 2-3 tsp. vanilla
>
> 1 cup warm water, not hot (I use milk to up the protein)
>
> 1 cup homemade mayonnaise

Mix the flour, sugar and baking powder. Add the baking soda to the warm water or milk. Add the warm, wet mix to the dry ingredients and mix with hand mixer. Add cocoa and fat, mix with mixer. Add mayonnaise and mix with mixer. Add vanilla

Bake for 45-60 minutes. Cake should be pulling from the edges of the pan, the kitchen should be filled with baked chocolate cake scents and a knife comes out clean when inserted in the center.

Vanilla Frosting

> 8 oz. package organic Neufchatel cheese
>
> 8 oz. container organic whipping cream
>
> 1 tbsp. maple syrup or raw, local honey
>
> 1 tbsp. vanilla

Place cheese in bowl and chop up. Add whipping cream, vanilla and maple syrup. Using hand mixer, blend until stiff enough for frosting a cake. Frost the mayonnaise cake when it cools and enjoy!

Paula M. Youmell, RN, MS, CHC

Chai Tea
(Very yummy with the breakfast puffs)

For 8 oz. mug:

¾ cup water

¼ cup milk

Cover and heat liquid slowly to a nice warm temperature, not boiling.

Add the following spices, have them measured out so you can add, stir and cover pot quickly:

¼ tsp. cardamom

¼ tsp. nutmeg

pinch of cloves

¼ tsp. ginger, rounded so it is a bit more than ¼

½ tsp. cinnamon (Ceylon cinnamon is best, cinnamon is actually cassia)

Optional: ¼ tsp. turmeric – this is a wonderful anti-inflammatory herb-spice. Try it, if you do not like the flavor it adds, leave it out.

Let steep for 5 minutes or so. Strain through a fine filter that will catch the powdered herbs.

Add ¼ tsp. real vanilla extract and ¼ to ½ tsp. raw, local honey and enjoy.

Other flavor extracts that are fun to play with instead of the vanilla: hazelnut, almond, coffee, chocolate. See what makes your taste buds happy while making your belly feel good!

If you have a sugar issue: high insulin from diabetic conditions, sugar addictions, yeast overgrowth, etc. Avoid the honey until you heal your condition.

Learn to play with recipes. Add more or less spices to suit your taste!

Apple Cider Vinegar Drink

>I cup water
>
>I tbsp. raw apple cider vinegar
>
>I tsp. raw, local honey

Mix together and drink.

You can add cayenne powder, from a pinch to a tsp. Cayenne is good for gut health.

"Egg Nog" Recipe

>I cup milk per person (nut and seed milks are good dairy substitutes, recipe below)
>
>I raw egg per cup of milk
>
>Spices: cinnamon, cardamom, nutmeg, ginger
>
>½ to I tsp. real vanilla per cup of milk
>
>¼ to ½ cup of cooked squash, sweet potato or yam per cup of milk (be brave and try cooked beet too!)

Put all ingredients in a blender and blend well. Spice to your taste, suggestions: cinnamon ¼ tsp. or more per cup of milk and a generous pinch of each nutmeg, ginger, and cardamom. Play with it. I also add sunflower seeds, walnuts, almonds in varying small amounts.

Caution: I need to remind you to use good, naturally-raised milk and eggs to avoid bacterial contamination from confined, animal factory farms.

Almond Milk

Put I cup of raw almonds (or other raw nut/seed) into 4 cups of water in a jar or dish you can cover tightly and let sit for 24 hours. You can make nut or seed milk without the soaking if you are in a hurry!

Stir or shake the jar on occasion. A ½ gallon, wide mouth, canning jar works well or cut the recipe in half and make in a quart size jar.

After 24-48 hours of soaking and shaking to soften and "sprouts" the almonds, throw it all in the blender and blend it like crazy. This is where a good blender is required. I love Vita Mix. Another good option, that is less pricey, is the Waring Pro Professional Quality Bar Blender.

Strain through a mesh strainer and store in the refrigerator. You can add vanilla and a little local raw honey or local maple syrup for flavor. Straining is not necessary, only if you want a "smoother milk." More nutrients and fiber are retained if you do not strain, just shake well before using.

If you have sugar addictions, blood sugar and/or insulin issues, yeast problems, high cholesterol... just use the vanilla! Skip the honey and maple syrup. The nut milk is yummy without being sweetened.

Cinnamon, cardamom, nutmeg, and ginger are yummy too!

You can use this basic recipe and make sunflower seed milk, walnut milk, sesame seed milk, any nut or seed that works in your diet! Peanuts are a bean, not a nut.

Chapter 11
Resources for Whole Health Living

Vegetarian Cookbooks

THIS IS A LIST OF the vegetarian cookbooks I have read and used over the years. My learning to cook vegetarian and vegan food made me a more creative and versatile cook. I can now grab random, fresh, local, seasonal produce and create delicious meals without recipes. It is a playful, fun, and creative process, much like art work to an artist. My canvas is the kitchen and food is my medium. May you become kitchen creative as well!

Moosewood Cookbook, Mollie Katzen

Vegan Nutrition Pure and Simple, Michael Klaper, MD

Fruit for All Seasons, Jennene Plummer

Field of Greens, Annie Somerville

Simply Vegan, Debra Wasserman

The Gradual Vegetarian, Lisa Tracy

The Green Door Restaurant Vegetarian Cookbook, Weaver, Poppy; Green Door Restaurant Staff

Uprisings, The Whole Grain Baker's Book, The Cooperative Whole Grain Educational Association

Home Bakebook of Natural Breads and Goodies, Sandra and Bruce Sandler

Home Gardener's Month By Month Cookbook, Marjorie Page Blanchard

From Asparagus to Zucchini, Madison Area CSA Coalition

Recipes from the Root Cellar, Andrea Chesman

This list is by no means exhaustive of all the available and wonderful vegetarian cookbooks to read and discover new foods, new techniques for cooking, and exciting, new flavors! I have also used ethnic cookbooks: Chinese, Thai, Indian, Native American, African, Southern American... the list goes on and on. Each one that I read (yes, like a novel) adds more color to my artistic cooking palette.

If the recipes include things like refined flours and sugars, I just replace them with whole food options. I also cut the sugar amount in a recipe by at least half. If a cake recipes calls for 2 cups of sugar, truthfully I never use more than ½ cup of sugar. I do the same for all baked goods. I then add extra vanilla and spices and you will never miss the hyper-sweetened baked goods!

The more versatile you become with cooking, the tastier and more entertaining your meals become. And the more you can enjoy your time in the kitchen "painting" with food! Have fun creatively cooking.

Movies to Explore

One of my favorite movies about healing is Andrew Weil's Spontaneous Healing. Dr. Weil is a gentle presence and he takes a wonderful and simple look at health and healing in this powerful movie.

Nutrition and food movies: If you type "Food Inc." into Netflix, you will get many recommendations for food, nutrition, and natural healing type movies. Here is a list that includes some of the many movies that have come out in the past few years around food, nutrition, health and healing. Use them as tools to find your own truth in this world of food, what works for you in regards to your personal health and healing within a whole food, whole health lifestyle. Enjoy!

Food, Inc.

Food Matters

Fresh

The Future of Food

King Corn: You Are What You Eat

Fat, Sick and Nearly Dead

Nourish (only 26 minutes and a very powerful movie!)

Supersize Me

Fast Food Nation

Sweet Misery (Aspartame)

Farmaggedon (Raw Milk Persecution)

Cancer, Nutrition & Healing

Keep seeking inspiring movies around food and nutrition, as more are being released all the time.

Book Recommendations

The books on health, healing, nutrition, food politics and economics are staggering. I will offer you suggestions to merely whet your appetite in the process of learning about your world, your body and how to heal. Read with pleasure in your heart, mind, and soul!

One of my favorite books on holistic health is The Male Herbal by James Green, Herbalist. I say this because the book has a profound way of moving you into the space of what holistic healing is truly about. I have used this book in many classes to help open peoples' minds to the possibility of healing, the possibility of caring for your body in something other than the "suppressing symptoms" method that is used almost exclusively by our current medical system. It is a great book for both males and females!

Susun Weed books:

Breast Cancer? Breast Health!

Wise Woman Herbal Healing Wise

Wise Woman Herbal Childbearing Year

Wise Woman Herbal New Menopausal Years

Down There

Rosemary Gladstar Books: a partial list

Family Herbal

Herbal Healing for Women

Rosemary Gladstar's Herbal Recipes for Vibrant Health

Food and Healing, Anne Marie Colbin

Whole Food Facts, Evelyn Roehl

the new whole foods encyclopedia, Rebecca Wood

Real Medicine Real Health, Dr. Arden Andersen

Beyond Antibiotics More than 50 Ways to Boost Immunity and Avoid Antibiotics, Schmidt, Smith and Sehnert

Sexual Nutrition, Dr. Morton Walker

Gut and Psychology Syndrome, Dr. Natasha Campbell-McBride, MD

Websites

There is an incredible number of food, nutrition, health and healing websites you can explore for hours! Once again, I recommend you read and find your own truth in all of this information. What works for one person does not necessarily work for everyone. I am only listing a couple of sites here as the number of websites is amazingly long.

http://www.mercola.com/

http://www.drweil.com/

http://www.susunweed.com/

http://www.sagemountain.com/

http://fiveelementsliving.com/

Retreat center owned, opening Fall 2013, by Shelby Connelly, L.Ac, located in beautiful Northern NY on the edge of the Adirondack Park. A restful haven for acupuncture, retreats… Create your own retreat and experience!

http://healthypets.mercola.com/

This website is for our pets, caring for them naturally just makes good sense.

http://www.thenaturalvet.net/ Another natural pet website. The "Bug Check" works wonders to keep fleas from infesting your pet or your home. I have used it very successfully. My only recommendation is that you need to give it to your pet every day if you want it to work. This means having a pet sitter giving it to your pet if you go away on summer vacations. If your loving pets are missing doses, the fleas will find them. Use as directed and you will be very happy with flea-free pets!

Products

Below I will list places to purchase body care, herbal and natural healing products. Once again, the list could be very long. I will give you companies I have used for years and trust.

http://www.mindseyefarm.com/

I list this one as Mind's Eye Farm is a local herb farm in my Northern NY area, making great teas and products. I recommend her teas: Calcium Comfort, Dandy Detox, North Country Mornings and North Country Nights. There are more, try them all! Order the tea blends in bulk! Try all the products under: Herbs for Mamas and their Babies, Herbs from our Kitchen, Herbal Medicine Cabinet, Bath and Beauty, and Herbal

Products for a Smooth Summertime. You will be delighted with the quality and performance of these products.

> http://www.aubrey-organics.com/ Body care, Aubrey Organics is my first and favorite love in the lotions, shampoos, and skin care products!
>
> http://www.eccobella.com/ Body care and cosmetics I love!

> http://www.drchristopher.com/

Herbal and natural products created by an amazing naturopathic healer, too many good ones to list them all!

> https://www.herbdoc.com/

Herbal nutritional supplements and healing products. Love the Superfood! We use it as our whole food vitamin!

> http://www.wisewomanherbals.com/

Herbal healing products. I have used many of these with clients, family, and friends. The products work!

> http://www.herbsetc.com/

I personally love the Deep Sleep gel caps. They are great for those nights when you just cannot get to sleep. I also whole heartedly recommend the Respiratonic and Lung Tonic. My second son was born three months premature. I chose to use these formulas to deal with his asthma and lung challenges from being premature. He never took any drugs or respiratory treatments despite some challenging problems. Ten years later his lungs are amazing! I have used the Para-Free to very successfully keep my many pets worm free. I use many of this companies formulas with my clients to address their health issues.

As I said, there are many excellent small companies making amazing natural products. Read labels on all body care, just because the front label claims the product is natural, it may actually be loaded with synthetic ingredients: Insist on truly natural. So read carefully; you deserve the best.

In regards to herbal products, research the company policy on the herbs they use in products. Are the herbs: organic, non-irradiated, environmentally and consciously wild crafted to preserve natural plants, and grown here in the USA? Ask how the company makes their products; do they create high quality strength products? Buy quality products as there are too many companies willing to make low quality products for their financial bottom line, not your whole health. Be a wise shopper and health consumer.

Bibliography or Lack Thereof!

Writer's Waiver: I write this book from the information in my head; you will not find a bibliography or footnotes. I have used my educational and real life experience as a registered nurse, school health and physical education teacher, yoga practitioner and teacher, herbalist, reiki practitioner, and whole food educator. I added the many dashes of wisdom I have gained through my holistic trainings under naturopaths, herbalists, energy healers, and many other natural healers, as well as the common sense that becomes inherent in working with the natural balance of life.

While I find true scientific research has its place in the world, I prefer to work from a space of common sense and rely on the natural world to guide me. I could be wrong, but I find that much research seems to be biased in the direction of the industry funding the research. I prefer nature.

For more information, go back and read My Preface and Disclaimer in the front of the book.

I hope you enjoyed our healing conversation. Go forward and create vibrant, whole health.

About the Author

Paula M. Youmell, RN, MS, CHC, is a NYS Registered Nurse and Licensed Health and Physical Education Teacher.

Paula's holistic certifications: Holistic Health, Nutrition and Fitness Educator, Certified Herbalist, Reiki Master. She enjoys putting her physical education knowledge to the task of teaching yoga classes to enhance the mind, body and soul connection.

Paula lives in northern NY State, hugging the Adirondack Park, with her two sons Jake and Eli, their dog and four cats. She loves Northern NY for the four seasons of outdoor activities: hiking, canoeing, biking, XC skiing, sledding, mountain climbing, camping...

Paula works as a private Holistic Health and Nutrition Consultant with individual clients, presents workshops in holistic health and healing, and teaches group classes in health, healing, and cooking.

www.HandsOnHealthHH.com
http://wholefoodhealer.wordpress.com/

Thanks for reading and contemplating whole health lifestyle changes!

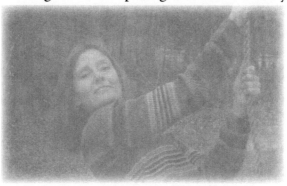

CPSIA information can be obtained at www.ICGtesting.com
Printed in the USA
BVOW08s0029240114

342840BV00002B/8/P